Phaco Fundamentals

A guide for trainee ophthalmic surgeons

Matthew Anderson and Jeremy Butcher

Matador
5 Weir Road
Kibworth Beauchamp
Leicester LE8 0LQ, UK
Tel: (+44) 116 279 2299
Fax: (+44) 116 279 2277
Email: books@troubador.co.uk
Web: www.troubador.co.uk/matador

ISBN 978-1848765-177

British Library Cataloguing in Publication Data.
A catalogue record for this book is available from the British Library.

Typeset in 11pt Sabon by Troubador Publishing Ltd, Leicester, UK

Matador is an imprint of Troubador Publishing Ltd

Contents

Acknowledgements

The authors gratefully acknowledge the support of Rayner Intraocular Lenses Ltd in the production of this book.

We also gratefully acknowledge the support of Leica, who contributed towards the illustrations in this book.

Diagrams and artwork by Jenni Ross and Jeremy Butcher.

Preface

Put at its simplest the modern cataract surgical procedure is the extraction of the diseased crystalline lens followed by the implantation of an artificial implant lens in its place. The cataractous lens is removed by phacoemulsification, a method introduced by Charles Kelman MD in the 1960s. Modern surgeons "do phaco" routinely and they inject intraocular lenses (IOLs) into the capsular bag with such apparent ease, yet forty years ago Kelman was struggling to persuade his contemporaries that phaco would work and the opposition he faced was just a fraction of the storm which Sir Harold Ridley endured from his peers to the IOL invention.

2009 is the 60th anniversary of the manufacture of Sir Harold's first IOL, which he implanted at St Thomas Hospital, London on 29th November 1949. That the two key steps – phacoemulsification and IOL implantation – have since then become so well established says much for the persevering spirits of the inventors and their alumni; but we should also pay tribute to the educationalists who painstakingly detailed their work, annotating step-by-step the evolution of lens extraction and IOL implantation procedures.

Without the teachers very little of that surgical expertise can be passed on to the next generation of cataract surgeons. Rayner, as the manufacturer of the first IOLs, worked closely with the great exponents of cataract microsurgery through the years and there is a long tradition in the company of support for the educational process of skills transfer; thus it is with great pleasure that we commend Dr Matthew Anderson and Mr Jeremy Butcher's clear and concise handbook on modern phacoemulsification techniques – confident that it will help many young surgeons to perform safe and successful cataract surgery through to the centenary year of the IOL in 2049.

Donald John Munro
Chairman and Managing Director
Rayner Intraocular Lenses Limited
(The manufacturer of the first IOL)

Foreword

As an Ophthalmology trainee you may be introduced to performing phacoemulsification surgery soon after commencing your first job, often with little previous microsurgical experience. Microsurgical skills courses go some way to addressing this problem, but these are necessarily intensive and cannot do much more than introduce some of the terminology and basic principles.

A potential problem with many surgical training systems is that your early learning experience may be highly dependent on

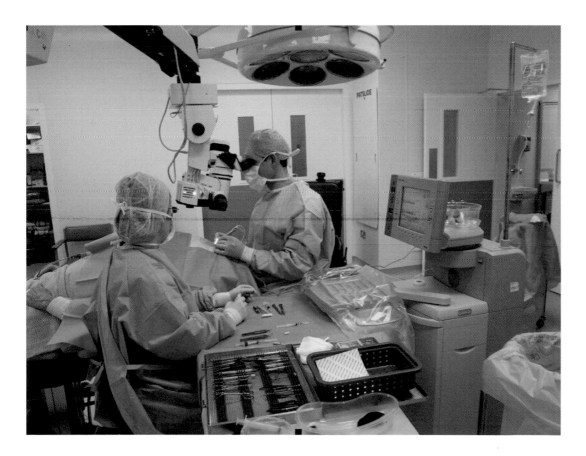

your supervising consultant. Some consultants will employ particular techniques which they have developed with years of experience because these make operating faster. However, such techniques may not be ideal or safe for you as a beginner if you have not yet acquired the necessary skills. Furthermore, attempting to start out emulating such supervisors can prove difficult and frustrating – you may even be unaware that alternative more conventional methods exist.

We saw the need for a concise, clear text which describes a *single safe way* to perform phacoemulsification surgery. This book aims to set out the principles and practical steps of such a method. We have deliberately omitted material that is not relevant to a junior trainee.

Descriptions of surgical steps are comprehensive and assume no prior knowledge of phacoemulsification surgery (although basic knowledge of ocular anatomy is required). The book is structured logically so that you can quickly find information most relevant to your immediate requirements in theatre.

We acknowledge that there are acceptable variations of most steps in phacoemulsification surgery, but feel it is important for learners to have a single safe method to which to refer. Throughout, justification is provided for the way particular steps are performed in our method.

In order to simplify explanations we have described surgery for a right-handed surgeon. We have intentionally avoided the subjects of anaesthesia, biometry and patient counselling – our focus is on the operative steps. We have not addressed the management of complications as this should be beyond the scope of a junior trainee.

There are many described ways of teaching/learning phacoemulsification surgery. These include repetition of a particular step before allowing progression to another, having a certain amount of time allocated for the trainee to operate, or allowing the trainee to perform the later steps of the operation before progressing to earlier ones. All have their merits – the choice will depend on your trainer.

Finally, there may be times when you lose confidence and feel that you will never reach that pinnacle of competence. Firstly, there is probably no true finishing point; the surgeon with insight will never achieve perfection. Secondly, the sensitive surgeon will continue to have crises of confidence throughout his/her career, although less commonly.

We hope that this book helps you on your way to performing safe, rewarding surgery.

1
Setting Up

You should visit the operating theatre prior to your first operating session in order to familiarise yourself with the equipment used in your unit, and to practise control of the operating microscope. *You must be competent in using the operating microscope before undertaking any intraocular surgery.*

Arrange a time when the theatre is free and familiarise yourself with the following:

The operating microscope

Most units use ceiling mounted microscopes (Fig 1.1), though features are similar for floor standing models.

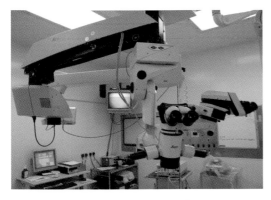

Fig 1.1 Ceiling mounted microscope

1. **Moving the microscope**
    You can manoeuvre the microscope manually by holding onto handpieces for this purpose (A, Fig 1.2). In some models it is necessary to rotate the handpieces first to disengage a brake mechanism which allows you to move it freely. Sterile plastic caps cover the handpieces during the operation.

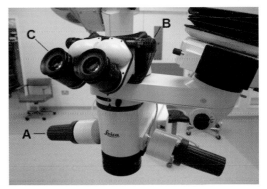

Fig 1.2 Microscope eyepiece mount

2. **Setting your Interpupillary Distance (IPD)**
    A knob situated on the eyepiece mount (B, Fig 1.2) allows you to adjust the distance between the eyepieces to match

your IPD. It is possible to measure your IPD by various techniques and dial in this value. However, we suggest simply looking down the microscope at a target and adjusting the IPD until you find the setting which gives you comfortable binocular vision

memorise this value for future reference

The knob should be covered with a sterile cap during each operation so that you can adjust the IPD intra-operatively (for example when changing positions with your supervising surgeon).

3. **Correcting for your refractive error**
   If you are ametropic you can adjust the eyepieces so that you can operate without spectacle correction. Simply rotate each eyepiece to dial in the dioptric value of your refractive correction.

   Alternatively set the eyepieces to zero and operate wearing your correction.

4. **Adjusting the angle of the eyepieces**
   You can adjust the angle that the eyepieces make with the horizontal by moving the eyepiece mount. If you feel more comfortable looking straight ahead while operating, position the eyepieces horizontally. If you prefer looking downwards, steepen the angle of the eyepieces.

5. **Spacers**
   Spacers (C, Fig 1.2) are adjustable plas-

tic extensions of the eyepieces. Their purpose is to help you to maintain a constant distance between your eyes and the eyepiece lenses when you operate without spectacles.

If you choose to use them, extend/pull out the spacers. In practice, many surgeons operate without spacers, leaving them unextended/pushed in.

6. **Control of the microscope footpedal**
   The footpedal is illustrated in Fig 1.3 and is operated with your left foot. It comprises at least three separate controls:

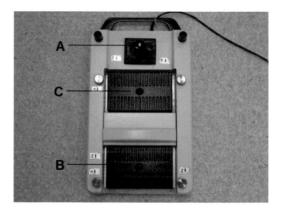

Fig 1.3 Microscope footpedal

i. *Joystick (A):* The joystick controls automated movement of the microscope in the XY (horizontal) plane; the microscope moves in the direction in which the joystick is pushed.

ii. *Magnification/Zoom (C):* This control is situated closest to you:

→ depressing one side of the pedal increases magnification and decreases field of view

→ depressing the other side of the pedal decreases magnification and increases field of view

iii. *Focus (B)*: This is situated between the joystick and the zoom control:

→ depressing one side of the pedal focuses up

→ depressing the other side of the pedal focuses down

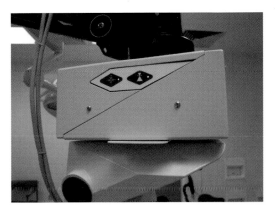

Fig 1.4 Buttons to centre the microscope; the green lights indicate it is centred

Practise using the above controls, observing a suitable target (e.g. a mannequin's eye) with the microscope. Appreciate that increasing the magnification not only decreases field of view, *but also decreases depth of field* (the antero-posterior distance which is in focus). This is important to bear in mind when you are attempting to gauge the depth of your instruments in the eye.

7. **Centering the microscope**
The microscope is centred before each operation by pressing the appropriate button (this is usually indicated by arrows such as > <) (Fig 1.4). This brings the instrument to the midpoint of its range of focus, its range of magnification, and its XY range. It ensures that at the commencement of the operation you will have a good range of focus, both up and down, a good range of zoom, both in and out, and a good range of travel in all directions in the XY plane.

8. **Adjusting the light intensity**
The brightness of the microscope's illuminating light can be adjusted on the light control panel (Fig 1.5). Most surgeons typically use an intensity of about 50% – you may vary this to suit your preference. The higher the intensity, the greater the potential risk of photo-stress retinal damage.

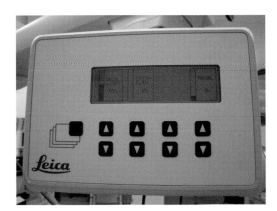

Fig 1.5 Light control panel

Setting a comfortable working position

It is *absolutely essential that you are comfortable* while operating. Discomfort, or even pain, caused by poor positioning/posture will interfere with your concentration and performance, which you can ill afford as a junior trainee.

The height of the microscope, the operating table and your chair can all be adjusted, as can the angle of the eyepieces. During your theatre visit set up the microscope, the table, the microscope footpedal and the phaco footpedal (see Fig 7.10) as if for a case. Place a mannequin's head (or other suitable target which would be at a patient's eye level) on the headrest of the operating table. Then experiment with adjusting all of the above until you find a combination where:

→ your feet easily reach the footpedals (but are not carrying your weight)

→ the target is in focus with the microscope centred

→ you can look down the eyepieces comfortably with your back straight

Note the heights of the chair and table (for example relative to your belt height), the

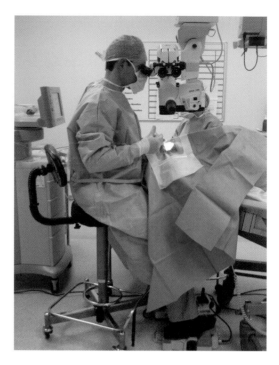

Fig 1.6 Correct operating position

angle of the eyepieces, and also the position of the footpedals relative to the head of the operating table, so that later you can quickly find your preferred working position.

(This step may sound unnecessary, but if omitted you may find yourself struggling to find a comfortable position the first time you are given an opportunity to operate. Not only does this not make a good impression, but with the operating team waiting you may feel pressured to accept a less-than-ideal operating position just to get underway... a poor start.)

Checklist

Before scrubbing up for a case, ensure that you have done the following:

- Set your IPD

- Corrected for your refractive error if appropriate

- Centred the microscope

- Positioned the patient, operating table, eyepiece angle, and footpedals to suit your preferences

- Set aside the chosen intra-ocular lens

- Administered an anaesthetic (if the surgery is not under general anaesthesia)

2
Draping

Eye and skin preparation

After scrubbing up, gowning and gloving, prep the eye and surrounding skin using 5% aqueous povidone-iodine (commercially available 10% solution should be diluted for ophthalmic use). In those allergic to iodine, chlorhexidine solutions are normally used. The area of skin which is prepped is shown in Fig 2.1.

- Use a folded swab held in sponge-holding forceps to apply the solution with the eye closed

    → be generous with the disinfectant solution, ensuring especially that the *eyelashes are thoroughly wet*

- Allow a small reservoir of solution to pool at the medial canthus and then ask the patient to open the eye, or lift the upper lid gently with the swab

    → this allows solution to run into the palpebral aperture onto the surface of the eye

    → it is useful to have a second

swab in position to prevent excess solution running down into the patient's ear

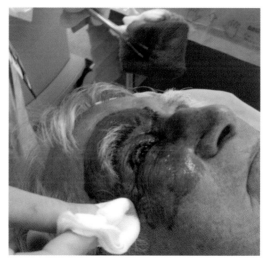

Fig 2.1 Eye and skin prepped with povidone-iodine

- Gently moving the upper lid with the swab ensures the disinfectant circulates to the fornices

    → remember that the bactericidal action requires time

- With the eye closed, dry the eyelids and surrounding skin with a dry swab held in sponge-holding forceps; start centrally and move progressively outwards in circular motions away from the eye; use a second dry swab if necessary

→ the *skin and lashes must be completely dry* to ensure that the drape adheres well

(In addition to prepping as described here, many surgeons instil drops of 5% aqueous povidone-iodine into the eye and onto the lashes prior to scrubbing up, after anaesthetising the eye. This allows about 5 minutes for a bactericidal effect.)

Draping

The most commonly used drapes are disposable. They have a central, transparent, adherent plastic window which is stuck down onto the skin surrounding the eye.

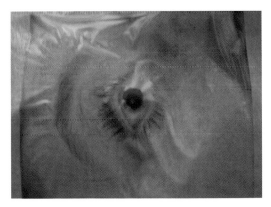

Fig 2.2 A disposable drape

- The drape is handed to you folded – observe the arrows/labels on the drape to confirm it is correctly orientated.

- Peel off the removable cover to expose the sticky surface of the window.

The next manoeuvre is illustrated in Fig 2.3:

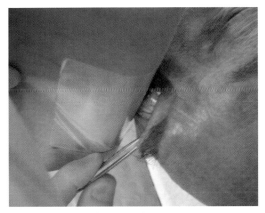

Fig 2.3 Elevation of the upper lid with forceps while applying the drape (surgeon's view)

- Ask the patient to look downwards – this will depress the lower lid if there is any residual muscle function after the anaesthetic.

- Use a pair of closed forceps to elevate the upper lid gently.

- Inform the patient that they will feel pressure on their face as the drape is stuck down in position.

- With the palpebral aperture now opened maximally, press the adherent portion of the *folded* drape down *onto the eye* **and periorbital skin** such that the centre of the window is positioned on the cornea

→ your aim when applying the

drape should be to *ensure that the eyelashes are stuck down away from the ocular surface* i.e. away from your surgical field (Fig 2.2)

- Ensure that the drape is adherent to the skin; press the plastic firmly against the skin.

- Unfold the drape → there are usually arrows on the drape indicating how it should be unfolded; take care not to touch the microscope, which should be positioned out of the way at this stage

  → ensure that where the drape covers the patient's nose and mouth, it is slightly tented upwards to leave room for comfortable breathing (Fig 2.4)

- The drape contains a plastic pouch into which excess irrigating fluid runs during the operation

  → open this pouch so that fluid can collect here

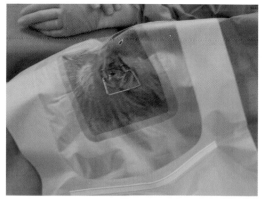

Fig 2.4 Drape in position, pouch opened

Inserting the eyelid speculum

The plastic window overlying the eye must now be cut and an eyelid speculum inserted:

- Use the fingers of your left hand to create tension in the plastic overlying the palpebral aperture if necessary.

- Open the blades of a pair of strabismus scissors and pierce the plastic overlying the medial canthus *carefully* with the tip of the lower blade.

- Cut towards the lateral canthus, along a line equidistant from the upper and lower lid margins (Fig 2.5)

  → ensure that you keep the lower blade well away from the cornea during the above manoeuvre

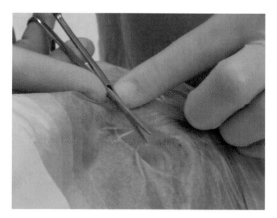

Fig 2.5 Cutting the drape

- In order for the drape to be stuck down properly in the region of the medial canthus, it is often necessary to make additional cuts in this region before pushing the plastic down onto the skin here.

- Use each arm of the speculum to fold the cut edges of the plastic drape into the upper and lower conjunctival fornices respectively, such that plastic now shields the surface of the eye from the lashes.

- Open the speculum widely to keep the lid margins away from the surgical field; the result is shown in Fig 2.6

    → your aim when inserting the eyelid speculum is to *keep the eyelashes away from the surgical field*

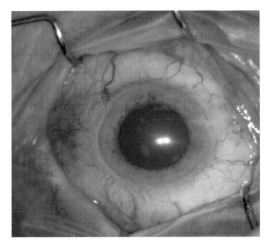

Fig 2.6 Speculum in position

3

The Corneal Section

You need to construct a self-sealing incision into the anterior chamber (AC) through the peripheral cornea near the limbus. This is usually performed at the 11 o'clock position, as in our method. Some surgeons always make the incision through temporal cornea, while others position it according to keratometry readings in an attempt to reduce pre-existing astigmatism.

Because the incision is small, you are unlikely to induce significant unwanted astigmatism.

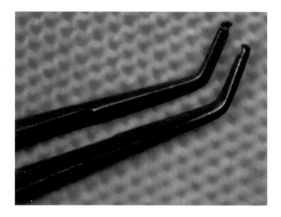

Fig 3.2 Notched forceps (Colibri forceps)

Instruments

The two instruments used are a keratome (Fig 3.1) and a notched forceps (Fig 3.2).

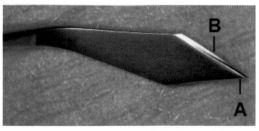

Fig 3.1 Keratome (see text: A = depth of blade at the end of step 1, B = depth at the end of step 2)

Method

The section/incision is made in three steps to create a multi-planar wound that is self-sealing. The result is depicted in Fig 3.3.

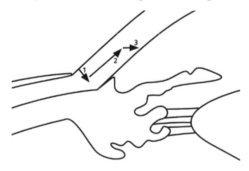

Fig 3.3 Construction of a 3-step corneal incision

All steps are performed under the micro-scope.

- Using the forceps, gently pick up the conjunctiva near the limbus at about the 11 o'clock position. Note how far the conjunctiva extends onto the cornea (Fig 3.4), before releasing it.

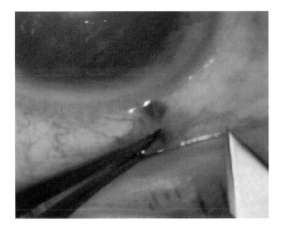

Fig 3.4 Determining the extent of the conjunctiva onto the cornea

You now use the forceps and keratome simultaneously to provide opposing forces as follows:

- With the forceps in your left hand, grasp the conjunctiva and underlying episclera at a point just peripheral to the planned incision site (Fig 3.6)

    → do not pick up the grasped tissue – simply rest the closed forceps gently on the underlying sclera

Step 1

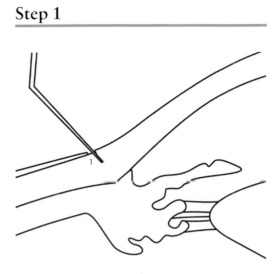

Fig 3.5 Step 1 of the corneal section

- Hold the keratome in your right hand, with the tip directed towards the centre of the eye.

- Enter the peripheral cornea just anterior to the conjunctival insertion identified earlier, at the 11 o'clock position (Fig 3.5 & 3.6).

- Advance the keratome such that the tip is just seen to enter the corneal stroma, then stop advancing

    → if you were not to provide any opposing force, the keratome would simply push the eye into depression rather than enter the cornea. Therefore exert *gentle* downwards pressure on the underlying sclera with the forceps to balance the force that you apply with the keratome

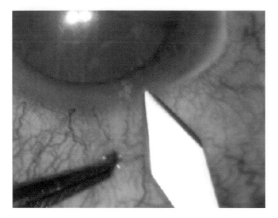

Fig 3.6 End of step 1

Step 2

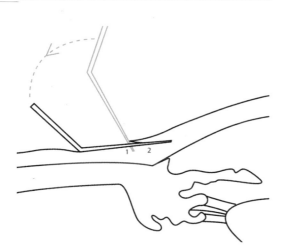

Fig 3.7 Step 2 of the corneal section

- With both instruments still in position, push the eye slightly into depression and then maintain the eye in this position (Fig 3.8) *(footnote)*.

- Flatten out the keratome blade, such that the heel of the blade rests on/slightly indents the underlying sclera (Fig 3.7)

→ the above two manoeuvres will render the blade almost parallel with the corneal epithelium and endothelium

- Advance the tip of the keratome for about 1.5mm, applying a counter force with the forceps as previously

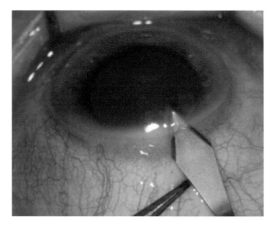

Fig 3.8 End of step 2 – note how the eye has been allowed into a depressed position

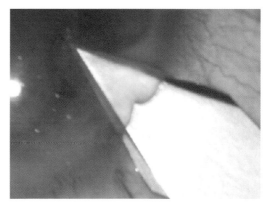

Fig 3.9 End of step 2

→ the tip of the keratome is still within the corneal stroma and has not yet entered the AC (Fig 3.9)

Step 3

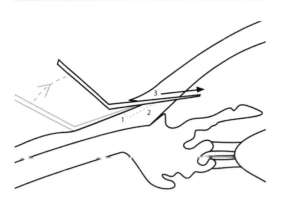

Fig 3.10 Step 3 of the corneal section

- Return the eye to the primary position.

- Adjust the angle that the keratome blade makes with the horizontal so that it is roughly parallel to the anterior capsule (Fig 3.10)

    → this manoeuvre will cause a depression in the cornea overlying the tip of the blade, associated with characteristic corneal stress lines (Fig 3.11)

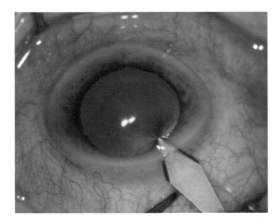

Fig 3.11 Corneal stress lines are seen near the tip of the keratome

- Advance the keratome into the AC, ensuring that the trajectory of the blade is *not too steep*, which may lead to the lens or iris being damaged, *or too flat*, which may cause damage to the corneal endothelium

    → the blade is advanced *only until its widest diameter* (the shoulders of the blade) *has just entered the AC*

    → the moment the shoulders of the blade enter the AC there will be no further resistance to the keratome. Therefore the *downward force applied with the forceps must be simultaneously relaxed* to prevent the eye being forced into elevation, causing the keratome to traumatize anterior segment structures

- Without delay, remove the keratome smoothly through the incision and release the forceps.

Note

Dividing construction of the corneal section into separate steps facilitates description, and it is useful to think of the steps while making the incision. However, you should aim to perform the section smoothly from start to finish, without pausing unnecessarily between steps.

Potential pitfalls

Incorrect incision length/angle

- Making step 1 too long may result in a full thickness stab incision. This may not self-seal.

- If you do not flatten out the blade sufficiently, you may enter the AC during step 2. This results in a 2-step incision which is less likely to self-seal.

- If you make step 2 too long, the seal of the wound around the instruments used later will be too tight. The result may be:

    → stress lines in the cornea near the wound when the instruments are in situ, distorting your view

    → a phaco burn: compression of the irrigation sleeve (chapter 7) by a tight wound leads to inadequate cooling and heat from the phaco probe damages the adjacent cornea, so that the wound is unlikely to self-seal

Incorrect angle when entering the AC

If you fail to keep the blade parallel to the anterior capsule during step 3, you may traumatize anterior segment structures.

Lingering in the AC

Once the shoulders of the keratome have entered the AC, aqueous leaks from the wound, shallowing the AC

→ if you leave the blade in the AC too long, you may inadvertently damage the anterior capsule as it moves forwards due to this shallowing

Helpful points

Throughout the operation your supervisor/scrub nurse will apply drops of BSS regularly to the cornea. This prevents drying of the epithelium and optimizes your view.

However, BSS should not be applied to the cornea immediately before you make the incision, as you should find it easier to perceive the depth of the blade in the stroma when the cornea is dry.

Footnote

Pushing the eye into slight depression brings the corneal epithelium and endothelium roughly parallel to the horizontal plane. This makes it easier for you to get the keratome blade parallel to these surfaces. If you leave the eye in the primary position you will have to angle the blade slightly up, which is more difficult.

4
The Paracentesis

Injection of viscoelastic

After you perform the corneal section, the AC will shallow due to loss of aqueous via the incision. It is important to refill the AC with a viscoelastic in order to restore its normal depth and architecture before proceeding further.

Viscoelastic

A viscoelastic is a pseudoplastic material. This means that its viscosity changes depending on its state of motion:

→ if it is stationary, as when left in the AC, it is more viscous, allowing it to keep the AC well-formed

→ if it is moving, as when being injected, it is less viscous, allowing it to pass through the narrow bore of a cannula

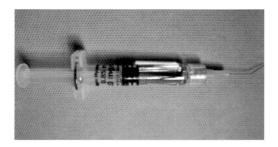

Fig 4.1 Cartridge of a viscoelastic loaded in a specially designed syringe

Method

- Accept a syringe filled with a viscoelastic and fitted with a blunt cannula.

- Prime the syringe before use in the eye by injecting just enough to form a drop of viscoelastic at the cannula tip – this ensures that all the air has been expelled.

- Under microscopic vision insert the cannula into the AC via the corneal section. Advance it to overlie the iris opposite the section

→ take care not to exert any

pressure on the anterior or posterior lips of the corneal section with the cannula

- Gently inject, observing the viscoelastic filling the AC. As it fills, withdraw the cannula gradually while still injecting, such that the AC is filled from the 5 o'clock position towards the 11 o'clock position.

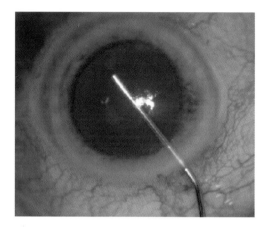

Fig 4.2 Filling the anterior chamber with a viscoelastic

- You will see aqueous humour being displaced and expelled via the corneal section as you inject.

- To know when the AC is full, observe the corneal section for the first sign of viscoelastic leaking from here, and then stop injecting.

Paracentesis

You need to create a small stab incision into the AC through the peripheral cornea near the limbus. This provides access for a second instrument during phacoemulsification. The incision is self-sealing.

Instruments

Instruments you use are the slit knife (Fig 4.3) and the notched forceps (Fig 3.2).

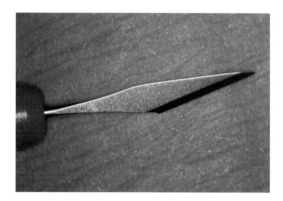

Fig 4.3 Slit knife

Method

- The paracentesis is typically made at the 2-3 o'clock position near the corneal limbus. Thus it is situated about $\frac{1}{4}$ of the corneal circumference away from the corneal section (the position may be varied slightly according to the second instrument you are using – your supervisor should advise you on the best site).

- Use the slit knife in your left hand, and the forceps in your right.

- Using the forceps, grasp the conjunctiva and episclera close to the limbus at about the 8-9 o'clock position i.e. opposite the site of the planned paracentesis (Fig 4.4)

→ do not pick up the grasped tissue, simply rest the closed forceps on the underlying sclera

Use the slit knife to make a stab incision as follows:

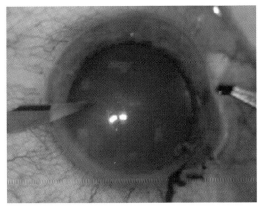

Fig 4.4 Performing the paracentesis

- Orientate the slit knife so that the blade is on its side, with the cutting edge facing away from you, as shown in Fig 4.4. Aim the tip of the blade *towards the centre of the anterior capsule*.

- Enter the peripheral cornea just in front of the conjunctival insertion (as for the corneal section)

  → as for the corneal section, you need to exert a counter force with the forceps. Push slightly towards the slit knife with the tips of the forceps to achieve this

- Advance the slit knife until about $1/3$ *of the length of the cutting edge has entered the AC.*

Take care not to damage the anterior capsule with the slit knife, especially if the AC is shallow → ensuring that the AC has been well formed with a viscoelastic reduces the risk of this.

- Withdraw the slit knife and release the forceps.

Note
The action with the slit knife is a *simple stab incision*. No sideways cutting action is used.

Potential pitfalls

Incorrect trajectory
If you angle the slit knife too steeply downwards you risk damaging the iris or anterior capsule. If you angle it upwards you may damage the corneal endothelium.

The trajectory of the slit knife must be towards the centre of the anterior capsule. This will match the desired trajectory for the shaft of the second instrument used later.

**Inserting the slit knife too far/
not far enough**

If you insert the slit knife too far you may traumatise the iris or anterior capsule.

If you fail to insert the slit knife far enough, the internal part of the corneal wound will be too small. The fit of the second instrument will be too tight, such that you may have difficulty inserting, removing or manoeuvring it.

5

The Capsulorhexis

In this step you tear a circular, central portion out of the anterior lens capsule, about 5mm in diameter (Fig 5.1). This yields a hole in the capsule, through which the lens will be removed.

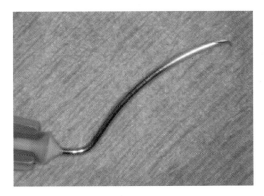

Fig 5.2 Pre-formed cystitome

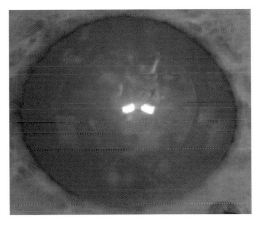

Fig 5.1 Completed capsulorhexis

Instruments

A cystitome either comes ready manufactured (Fig 5.2), or is made by modifying a 28 gauge needle (Fig 5.3), as described below.

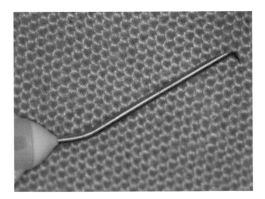

Fig 5.3 28 gauge needle modified to form a cystitome

You also use a capsulorhexis forceps.

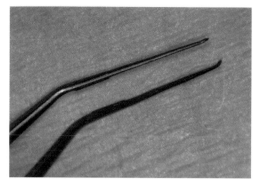

Fig 5.4 Capsulorhexis forceps

- Ensure that the anterior chamber is fully filled with a viscoelastic.[1]

- You may find increasing the magnification helpful.

- Focus down so that the *anterior capsule is perfectly in focus.*

Preparing a cystitome needle

- Accept a 28 gauge needle mounted on a 2ml syringe, containing either Balanced Salt Solution (BSS) or viscoelastic.

- Under the microscope, use a needle holder to bend firstly the bevel of the needle, and secondly the shaft of the needle (as shown in Fig 5.5 & 5.6), in such a way as to produce the desired result.

Performing the capsulorhexis

Creating a flap
- Hold the syringe containing BSS or viscoelastic, mounted with the cystitome, in your right hand; you may find it helpful to use your left hand to provide extra stability.

- Under the microscope, insert the cystitome into the anterior chamber through the corneal section

    → insert the tip on its side so as

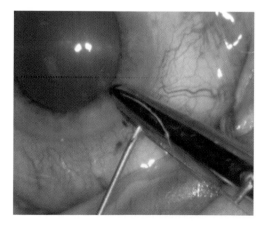
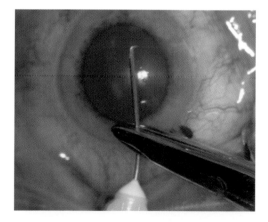

Fig 5.5 & 5.6 28 gauge needle bent to form a cystitome using a needle holder

not to traumatize the wound

→ try not to exert any pressure on the wound margins during this manoeuvre to avoid leakage of viscoelastic

• Now point the cystitome tip towards the anterior capsule and bring it to overlie the centre of the capsule.

• Tilt the cystitome so that the tip *just pierces* the anterior capsule

→ *in doing this, use the corneal section as a pivot point, without pushing down on the floor of the corneal wound*

• Keeping the needle tip at the same depth (i.e. just piercing the capsule), start moving it peripherally towards point A, as shown in Fig. 5.7 *(footnote)*

→ you will see a tear developing in the anterior capsule

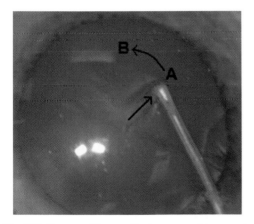

Fig 5.7 The cystitome tip is moved towards 8 o'clock while just piercing the anterior capsule, creating a tear

→ if the needle tip sinks too deeply into the lens during this manoeuvre, the cortex will be disrupted and the tear will become more difficult to see against the red reflex

• After extending the tear as far as point A shown in Fig 5.7, begin moving the cystitome tip in an arc towards point B

→ gently continuing this movement will cause the tear to propagate in the direction of B

→ this is the start of the circumferential tear which will form the capsulorhexis

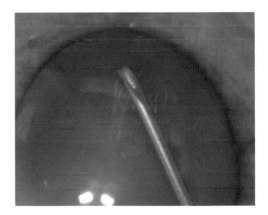

Fig 5.8 Moving the tip as described causes the tear to propagate circumferentially

→ an elevated flap of anterior capsule results

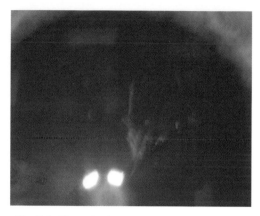

Fig 5.9 Elevated capsular flap is formed

The distance you move peripherally (i.e. the location of point A) before beginning the arc towards B in part determines the size of the capsulorhexis.

- If necessary, use the needle tip to elevate the free edge of the flap slightly off the underlying cortex, so that you will be able to grasp it with the forceps in the next step.

- Remove the needle from the AC with the tip on its side.

Leading the tear around

- ***Ensure that the AC is still well filled with viscoelastic*** – refill it if necessary.[1]

- Hold the capsulorhexis forceps in your right hand; again your left hand may provide stability.

- Insert the closed forceps into the AC

through the corneal section, without distorting the wound.

- Use the forceps to grasp the free edge of the flap cleanly, without touching the cortex. Then move in an arc in the direction shown in Fig 5.10

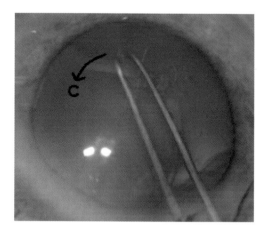

Fig 5.10 Grasp the free edge of the elevated flap. Move in an arc towards C

→ the capsulorhexis tear will be propagated in this direction. The result will be similar to that shown in Fig 5.11

→ note that the flap has now lengthened. Because of this the forceps tips will be further from the leading/evolving edge of the capsulorhexis

- To maintain good control of the direction of the tear, release the forceps from the flap and *regrasp the free edge at a point closer to the leading edge* (Fig 5.11 & 5.12).

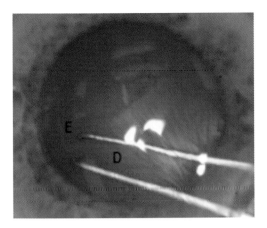

Fig 5.11 Approximately ¼ of the rhexis completed. Release the forceps from D and regrasp at E, closer to the leading edge

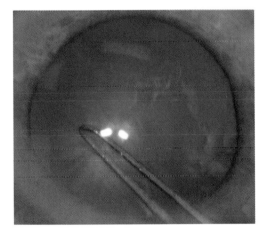

Fig 5.12 Regrasping the flap closer to the leading edge

- You are now ready to continue the rhexis/tear.

Your objective is to create a circular hole in the anterior capsule as shown in Fig 5.1.

This is done by grasping the flap close to the leading edge, applying the appropriate force with the forceps so that the tear extends a short distance in the desired direction, releasing the flap and regrasping it closer to the leading edge, and so on.

Key principles

It is not possible to describe adequately the vectors that must be applied to complete the capsulorhexis – a feel for this must be acquired by practising tearing a rhexis in a sheet of cellophane, or better still in a Wet Lab session.

However, the key principles which apply are as follows:

- When the flap is grasped close to the leading edge, the tear will tend to follow the direction of the forceps tips.

- The longer the flap extends before you regrasp it, the less control you have. *Therefore we suggest that you regrasp the flap frequently during the rhexis i.e. before it extends more than ¼ of the circumference of the final capsulorhexis.*

- Directing the forceps away from the pupil centre (centrifugally) causes the tear to extend outwards, towards the equator.

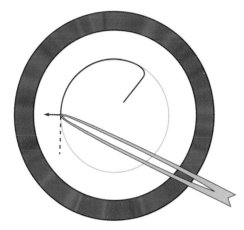

Fig 5.13 A more centrifugal vector applied with the forceps causes the rhexis to be directed outwards

- Directing the forceps towards the centre of the pupil (centripetally) causes the tear to be directed inwards, away from the equator

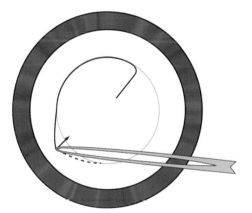

Fig 5.14 A more centripetal vector applied with the forceps causes the rhexis to be directed inwards

→ *if the capsulorhexis begins to extend too peripherally, you must apply a more centripetal vector*

As you lead the capsulorhexis around, observe its progress and adjust the amount of centripetal/centrifugal force you are exerting as necessary.

Potential pitfalls

Incorrect size of capsulorhexis
Endeavour to make your capsulorhexis about 5mm in diameter. Bear in mind that pupil dilatation will vary considerably from patient to patient, so *you should not use the distance from the pupillary margin to guide the size of your rhexis.*

Rhexis too large
Starting the circumferential tear too peripherally, or exerting too much centrifugal force during the rhexis, will lead to a capsulorhexis that is too large.

The problems with a large rhexis are:

- the leading edge is closer to the equator. Therefore if the rhexis starts to tear outwards, there is less room for you to take corrective action. If the rhexis tears outwards from a position that is already fairly peripheral, it may extend to the equator

- a large capsulorhexis makes it more likely for the lens to prolapse forwards out of the capsular bag during hydrodissection (Chapter 6)

Rhexis too small
If you are not peripheral enough when you start the circumferential tear, or if you exert too much centripetal force during the rhexis,

the resulting capsulorhexis will be too small.

The problem with a small rhexis is that you have a smaller area through which to remove the lens matter in subsequent steps.

Rhexis extending peripherally/tearing out

If you fail to exert the correct vectors with the forceps, or if there is significant loss of viscoelastic via the section[1], you may find the rhexis tearing out towards the equator.

If this happens, <u>STOP</u>.

Refill the AC completely with viscoelastic. Grasp the flap again and pull directly towards the centre of the pupil i.e. exert a purely centripetal force

> → this should lead the tear inwards

Subincisional rhexis

You may find it difficult to see the leading edge in the 12 o'clock to 10 o'clock sector. This is because your view is partly obstructed by the forceps and may be partly obscured by corneal stress lines

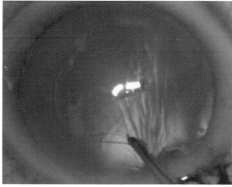

Fig 5.15 Corneal stress lines distorting the subincisional view

> → minimise corneal distortion by pivoting the forceps in the wound and not pressing on the wound margins

It is best not to have to regrasp the flap in this area:

> ＞ make sure that you regrasp the flap just before reaching this area so that you won't need to do so here

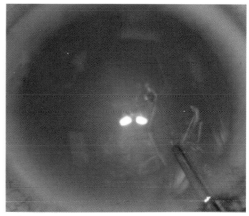

Fig 5.16 Leading the rhexis through the subincisional region

Helpful points

• Sometimes the flap becomes folded on itself, such that the free edge becomes difficult to see. Injecting viscoelastic close to the flap will move it, possibly making it easier to see the edge.

• Avoid grasping a fold of the capsular flap, such that two layers of capsule are held by the forceps, as this affords you less control.

Rationale

[1] Fig 5.17 shows that shallowing of the AC, as occurs if viscoelastic leaks from the section, results in a greater tendency for the rhexis to extend peripherally.

Footnote

Moving towards the 8 o'clock position means that when the flap is raised, it aligns well with the long axis of the forceps, making it easy to grasp.

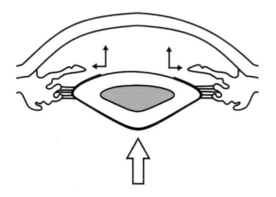

Fig 5.17 Effect of AC shallowing on vectors at the leading edge

6
Hydrodissection

In this step you inject a jet/wave of BSS to cleave the lens cortex from the surrounding lens capsule, so that the lens may be freely rotated later during phacoemulsification.

Instruments

Use a 2ml syringe filled with BSS, mounted with a narrow gauge blunt cannula (e.g. Helsinki cannula).

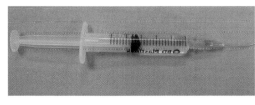

Fig 6.1 Syringe mounted with hydrodissection cannula

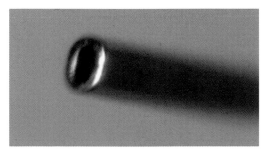

Fig 6.2 Flattened profile of a hydrodissection cannula

Method

- Prime the syringe, ensuring all air is expelled. Hold it in your right hand, using your left hand for additional support if necessary. The concave curve of the cannula faces upwards.

- Under the microscope, insert the cannula into the AC via the corneal section, avoiding pressure on the wound margins.

- Focus the microscope on the lens surface and capsulorhexis.

- Advance the cannula to a point just overlying the lens cortex, immediately in front of the free edge of the capsulorhexis, opposite the corneal section (i.e. at the 5 o'clock position).

The cannula must now be advanced just beneath the free edge of the anterior capsule (Fig 6.3 & 6.4).

- To accomplish this, first move the tip of the cannula very gently downwards – in a routine case the lens cortex is soft enough to allow this manoeuvre to cause the cannula to indent the surface of the cortex minimally

→ this brings the cannula tip to a level *just deep to the capsule's free edge*

• Now advance the cannula tip about 0.5mm peripherally under the edge of the capsule. You should be able to see that the cannula is clearly beneath the anterior capsule (gently lifting the tip will cause the capsule to tent anteriorly, confirming that it is beneath the capsule).

Principles guiding hydrodissection

• Injection of BSS now will cause a jet of fluid to strip the lens cortex from the capsule progressively (Fig 6.3). This will commence at the cannula tip and proceed around the equator and behind the lens

→ you can usually see the wave of injected BSS clearly against the red reflex as it progresses around the back of the lens (Fig 6.4a-c). *Observation of this fluid wave* is an indication that some hydrodissection has occurred

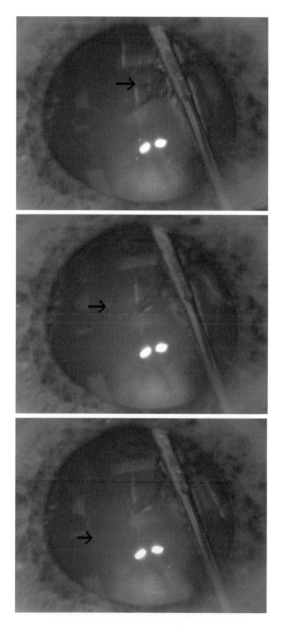

Fig 6.4a-c As you inject BSS, a fluid wave progresses around the back of the lens

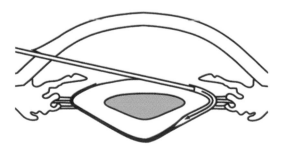

Fig 6.3 Injection of BSS cleaves cortex from the capsule

→ a second, more subtle sign that hydrodissection has occurred is a slight forwards/anterior movement of the lens. Look out for this, as sometimes it is not possible to see a fluid wave

- We recommend repeating this step at a minimum of two additional sites to ensure that the lens is well hydrodissected and will rotate easily later during phacoemulsification

  → advance the cannula beneath the anterior capsule at about the 3 and 8 o'clock positions respectively and repeat the above step. You *may* see additional fluid waves when BSS is injected at these sites

- The force of injection and amount to be injected can only be learned by experience, but useful principles are:

  → initially inject gently and constantly. Depending on the observed result you may need to increase the force of injection.

  If you see a wave developing, continue injecting gently until it has progressed *all the way* around the back of the lens

  → sometimes, despite correct technique, you may not see either a fluid wave or forward movement of the lens when you inject at the initial site. Rather than continuing to increase the force of injection, move to one of the additional sites and try hydrodissection there. Usually one of the sites will prove successful

  → the amount of BSS that needs to be injected is variable. Once you have seen a fluid wave progress all the way around behind the lens there is no need to inject further at that particular site, but bear in mind that a wave will not always be seen

It is important to realise that subsequent steps are dependent on your hydrodissection. A thorough hydrodissection makes later steps much easier.

Prolapse of the lens

It is fairly common for thorough hydrodissection to cause the lens to begin to prolapse forwards out of the capsular bag (Fig 6.5) – this often happens following injection at the 2nd or 3rd site.

Should this occur, prevent complete prolapse out of the bag as follows:

- Lie the shaft of the cannula horizontally across the surface of the lens (Fig 6.6).

- *Gently* push it backwards.

- If part of the lens does prolapse out of the bag (Fig 6.7), you can usually reposition it in the bag by performing the above manoeuvre.

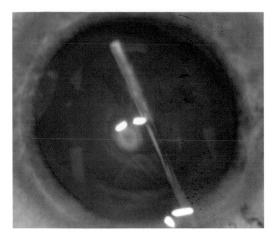

Fig 6.5 Lens beginning to prolapse at the 7 o'clock position

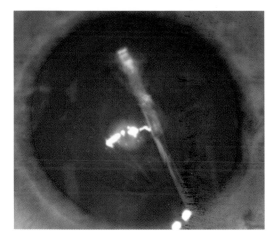

Fig 6.6 Pushing downwards with the cannula to prevent lens prolapse or to reposition the lens in the capsular bag

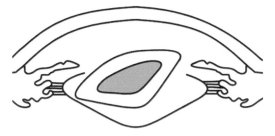

Fig 6.7 Prolapse of part of the lens out of the capsular bag

Note

After hydrodissection some surgeons attempt to rotate the lens within the capsular bag to confirm adequate hydrodissection.

We do not perform this step for the following reasons:

→ the vectors required to exert a purely rotational force on the lens are most easily applied using grooves formed later during phacoemulsification; attempting to rotate the lens without using these grooves exerts forces other than purely rotational ones, placing unnecessary strain on the zonules

→ if attempts at rotation later using the grooves reveal hydrodissection to be inadequate, additional hydrodissection can be performed at that stage

Hydrodelamination

This is similar to hydrodissection, but here you inject a jet/wave of BSS to create a cleavage plane within the epinucleus all the way around the nucleus (Fig 6.9). Advantages of performing hydrodelamination are:

→ during phacoemulsification later (see chapter 8), the nuclear quadrants can be removed independently of epinuclear lens matter.

The epinucleus which remains behind 'splints' the posterior lens capsule during removal of the nuclear quadrants, preventing the capsule (PC) from moving forwards towards the phaco-tip

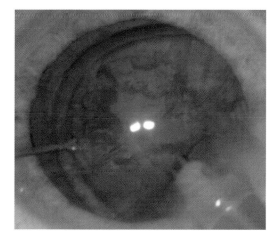

Fig 6.8 If hydrodelamination is performed, epinucleus remains in the capsular bag after removal of the nucleus

→ hydrodelamination may facilitate rotation of the nucleus later (chapter 8), complementing hydrodissection

Method

- If you choose to perform hydrodelamination, do this immediately after hydrodissection, without removing the cannula.

- Position the tip of the cannula just overlying the lens cortex, immediately

in front of the free edge of the anterior capsule, opposite the corneal incision at about the 5 o'clock position (i.e. the same as when commencing the hydrodissection).

- Gently move the cannula tip downwards/posteriorly so that it penetrates the lens cortex, and advance it about 1mm in a downwards and peripheral direction. The tip is now embedded within the epinucleus (Fig 6.9).

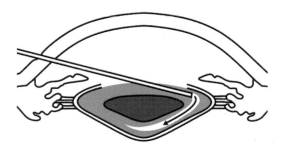

Fig 6.9 Hydrodelamination creates a cleavage plane within the epinucleus

- Inject *gently* → this creates a cleavage plane within the epinucleus which progresses around behind the nucleus.

- If hydrodelamination is successful you may observe the 'golden ring sign', where the cleavage plane creates a halo effect (Fig 6.10)

  → note that *only adequate hydrodissection is essential.* Frequently you will not obtain a convincing golden ring sign – as long as you consider your hydrodissection to be adequate do not struggle unnecessarily to obtain evidence of hydro-delamination

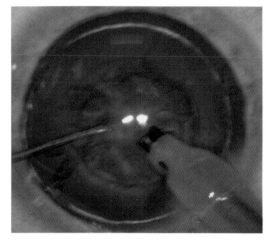

Fig 6.10 Golden ring sign

Potential pitfalls

Subincisional hydrodissection
The cortical lens matter in the subincisional region is usually the most difficult to cleave from the capsule. Inadequate hydrodissection in this region is a frequent cause of difficulty in rotating the lens later during the operation (chapter 8).

Strategies to deal with this problem include:

Prevention
Ensure that you see a convincing fluid wave progressing *all the way* around the back of the lens. Injecting at multiple sites improves hydrodissection.

The J-cannula
This cannula can be used to hydrodissect

by injecting fluid under the subincisional anterior capsule, as shown in Fig 6.11. The fluid wave thus progresses in the opposite direction to the conventional method. This technique facilitates cleavage of cortex from capsule in the subincisional region.

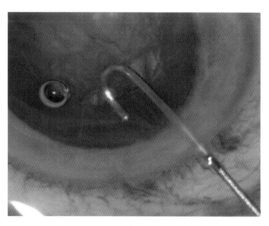

Fig 6.11 Use of the J-cannula

You may choose to use both types of cannula to hydrodissect. This results in thorough hydrodissection, but with a resultant tendency for the lens to prolapse at the end of the hydrodissection

→ therefore start with the J-cannula. If the lens begins to prolapse later when you are completing the hydrodissection with the straight cannula, this can more readily be used to push it backwards as described previously

Hydrodissection via the paracentesis
It is possible to perform hydrodissection in the subincisional area with a straight cannula via the paracentesis. This is not

described further as this technique should be beyond the scope of a junior surgeon.

Soft cataracts

Soft cataracts are more difficult to hydrodissect. They are also more difficult to rotate (chapter 8). Therefore inject at multiple sites and try to obtain more than one fluid wave to ensure complete hydrodissection.

7

Phaco Equipment and Settings

This chapter aims to provide you with a basic working knowledge of phacoemulsification equipment and the various settings which are commonly used.

The phaco handpiece

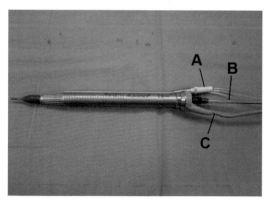

Fig 7.1 The phaco handpiece

The phaco tip

The phaco handpiece/probe contains a hollow metal needle which ends in a bevelled tip (Fig 7.2). This is made of titanium alloy.

When phaco power is applied, the tip of the needle oscillates back and forth at a very high frequency (± 40 kHz). This action:

i) physically emulsifies (smashes up) hard nuclear lens matter if it is in contact with the tip. This enables you to aspirate it

ii) causes cavitation, an effect whereby high pressure and temperature are generated in front of the tip. Cavitation emulsifies lens matter immediately ahead of the tip, even if it is not in contact with the tip

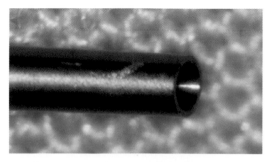

Fig 7.2 The phaco needle (irrigation sleeve removed)

The amount of phaco power delivered is determined by the amplitude of travel of the phaco tip → a greater amplitude results in more power.

Lens matter is aspirated through the hollow core of the needle.

The irrigation sleeve

A plastic sleeve covers most of the phaco needle. Irrigation fluid circulates under this sleeve, cooling the needle. The irrigation fluid then leaves via two irrigation ports on opposite sides of the needle (Fig 7.3).

The sleeve is twisted into place on the phaco probe, and can be adjusted such that the amount of needle tip exposed beyond the sleeve can be varied. You must ensure that the correct amount of exposed needle is showing before inserting the probe into the eye

> → Fig 7.3 shows approximately the correct amount of needle tip exposed beyond the irrigation sleeve

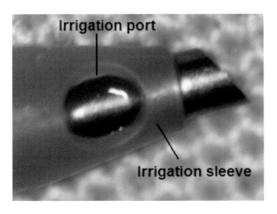

Fig 7.3 Correct amount of needle exposed beyond the sleeve

→ Fig 7.4 shows too little tip exposed: you would not be able to get a good view of the end of the needle tip during phacoemulsification, as it would be hidden by the sleeve. Also, there would not be enough exposed tip to groove effectively with each stroke. Therefore twist the sleeve anti-clockwise to expose more needle

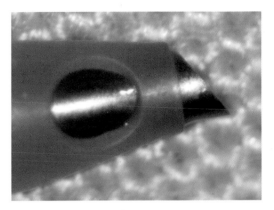

Fig 7.4 Too little phaco needle exposed beyond the sleeve

→ Fig 7.5 shows too much needle exposed: this results in the tip being too far from the irrigation ports. As a result, when you first insert the needle tip into the AC, the irrigation ports might not reach the AC but end up positioned within the corneal section. Therefore twist the sleeve clockwise to reduce the amount of exposed tip.

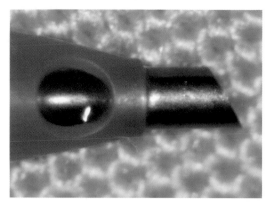

Fig 7.5 Too much needle exposed beyond the sleeve

Positioning of the irrigation ports
When the probe is held with the bevel facing upwards, the irrigation ports must be directed to each side (Fig 7.3)

→ if, when twisting the sleeve into place, the ports are mistakenly aligned such that one of them points upwards (Fig 7.6), irrigation fluid will be directed onto the corneal endothelium during phaco, causing unnecessary stress on the tissue

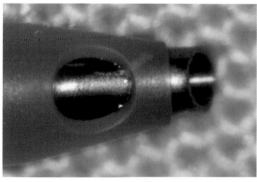

Fig 7.6 INCORRECT alignment of the irrigation ports

The piezo-electric crystal
The phaco handpiece contains a piezo-electric crystal. When an alternating electric current is passed through the crystal, it rapidly expands and contracts → this is the mechanism which causes the phaco needle to oscillate back and forth.

When phacoemulsification power is activated, the handpiece emits a high-pitched rasping sound which is easily audible.

The phaco handpiece lines

See Fig 7.1

<u>Line A</u>: The irrigation line carries irrigating fluid to the handpiece

<u>Line B</u>: The aspiration line carries aspirated fluid away from the handpiece

<u>Line C</u>: The electrical supply to the handpiece

The phaco machine

The controls and displays of your phaco machine may differ from those described here. You should familiarise yourself with the machine used in your unit.

See Fig 7.7

A – Visual Display Unit & keypad
These are operated by the assisting nurse according to your instructions.

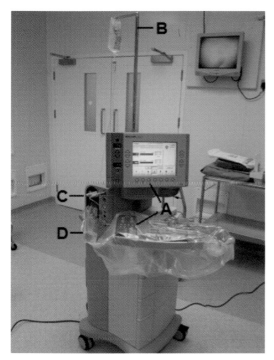

Fig 7.7 Phaco machine

The screen indicates the various settings and modes that are in use. Changes are made via touch screen controls or a keypad control, which are covered by sterile transparent drapes. Many control systems give audio confirmations of changes, which you should listen out for after requesting a setting to be altered.

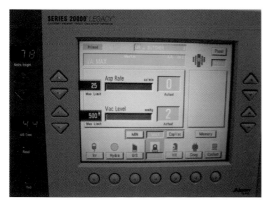

Fig 7.8 Visual Display Unit

Further details are not given as each make of machine will differ in screen displays and controls. You should familiarise yourself with the machine used in your unit.

B – The bottle arm

The bottle/bag containing the irrigation fluid is suspended from a metal arm, the height of which can be adjusted. Surgeons typically ask for 'bottle up' or 'bottle down'.

The irrigation fluid flows purely under the force of gravity, so adjusting the height relative to the eye alters the infusion pressure.

C – The peristaltic drive

The mechanism by which suction is created to aspirate fluid depends on the type of phaco machine. Peristaltic and Venturi systems are the two most widely used. We describe dynamics and settings for a peristaltic machine.

Fig 7.9 shows a peristaltic drive. Fluid is essentially milked along by rollers which compress the tube. The speed with which the rollers turn determines the requested aspiration rate.

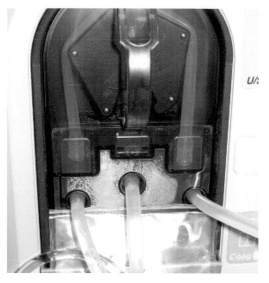

Fig 7.9 The peristaltic drive

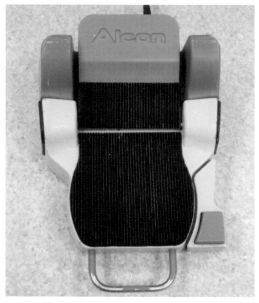

Fig 7.10 The phaco footpedal

D – Fluid reservoir
Aspirated fluid collects in a disposable plastic bag at the side of the phaco machine.

The footpedal

Irrigation, aspiration and phacoemulsification power are all controlled via the phaco footpedal. The same footpedal is used to control irrigation and aspiration during the 'I/A' (irrigation/aspiration) step of the operation (chapter 10).

Most surgeons operate the footpedal with their right foot.

The pedal can be successively depressed into three different positions:

Position 1
When you begin to depress the pedal, the first position you engage is Position 1. This activates irrigation

→ as irrigation is activated you may hear a click as a pinch valve releases in the phaco machine, allowing the flow of irrigating fluid

→ you will see fluid flowing out of the irrigation ports

The click of the valve may also be heard when you stop irrigating i.e. disengage Position 1.

Depressing your foot further within Position 1 (i.e. the green zone in Fig 7.11) *does not alter the rate* of irrigation, which is determined by the bottle height and the resistance to flow in the system.

Position 2
Depressing the pedal further engages

Position 2, activating aspiration as well as irrigation. This is signalled by a constant sound from the phaco machine.

Usually the machine is programmed such that depressing the pedal further within Position 2 causes a higher rate of aspiration. The relationship between depression of the pedal and the aspiration rate is usually programmed to be linear.

If you return to Position 1 aspiration stops, leaving only irrigation active.

Position 3
When you depress the phaco pedal still further you will engage Position 3, activating phacoemulsification power as well as irrigation and aspiration. A high-pitched sound is emitted from the handpiece while phaco power is active.

Depressing the pedal within Position 3 generates increased phaco power, usually in a linear relationship. The intensity of the handpiece sound output increases with increased power.

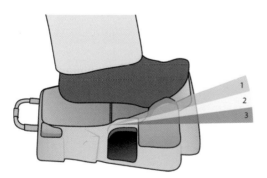

Fig 7.11 Phaco footpedal positions: Position 1: irrigation only; Position 2: irrigation + aspiration; Position 3: irrigation + aspiration + phaco power

Returning to Position 2 stops phaco power, leaving aspiration and irrigation active.

Continuous irrigation
Sometimes it is useful to activate continuous irrigation, such that fluid is constantly infused without you having to keep the pedal in Position 1. (This is especially useful during the I/A step of the operation (chapter 10) if you find that you have a tendency to disengage Position 1 inadvertently, resulting in shallowing of the AC.)

Tapping the control labelled X (Fig 7.12) to the right with your foot activates continuous irrigation *(footnote)*. An audible signal is heard as this engages. You can still use the pedal as usual to engage other footpedal positions. If you want to stop continuous irrigation tap the same control to the right again.

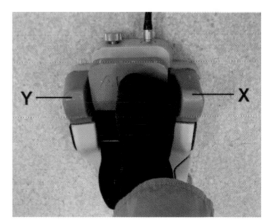

Fig 7.12 Activating/deactivating continuous irrigation

Reflux
It may be necessary to cause reflux of fluid from the aspiration port during I/A (chap-

ter 10), for example if posterior capsule is aspirated accidentally.

Tap control Y (Fig 7.12) to the left with your foot to cause a short burst of refluxed fluid. Only a short burst results – you do not have to tap it again to stop regurgitation of fluid *(footnote)*.

Settings

Aspiration
Fluid or lens matter is sucked up the hollow tip of the phaco needle or the aspiration port of the I/A handpiece (chapter 9), travels via the aspiration line and collects in a bag at the side of the phaco machine.

Aspiration causes mobile lens fragments to be sucked towards the tip of the handpiece.

The *requested* aspiration rate is determined by the amount that you depress the phaco pedal within Position 2. The *actual* resultant aspiration rate is determined also by other factors, such as the degree of occlusion of the phaco tip or I/A aspiration port and the viscosity of fluid being aspirated.

The maximum achievable rate by complete pedal depression within Position 2 is programmable. This is typically set between 18 – 45 ml/min, depending on the stage of the operation (see later).

Vacuum
If the phaco tip or the I/A aspiration port

is occluded by lens matter while you are aspirating, vacuum will result behind the occlusion (this applies to a peristaltic type machine).

This vacuum is essentially a force which allows you to hold onto and move lens matter which is occluding the tip.

Vacuum can be increased by increasing the rate of aspiration while the tip/port is occluded. A *maximum achievable vacuum* is programmable to prevent unnecessary and dangerous levels of vacuum from being generated. Maximum settings vary from 0mmHg to about 400mmHg, depending on the stage of the operation.

The pitch of the machine's audio output rises with increasing vacuum → you can therefore gauge the vacuum level by paying attention to the sound.

Irrigation
Irrigation fluid travels from the bottle/bag, down the irrigation line and into the eye via the irrigation ports near the tip of the phaco probe or I/A probe.

This is *purely gravity driven*. The rate of irrigation is determined by the height of the bottle relative to the eye and the resistance to flow in the system. *The bottle height is usually between 65cm and 105cm above the patient's eye level.*

The resistance to flow is in turn determined by factors such as the length and diameter of inflow tubing and the type of phaco needle and sleeve.

Phaco power

Phaco power determines the ability of the oscillating tip to emulsify hard nuclear matter.

Power is increased by depressing the pedal within Position 3. The *maximum achievable power* with full pedal depression is programmable. It is typically *expressed as a percentage of the power that the machine is capable of producing*

> → thus a *typical power setting of 60%* means that if you fully depress the pedal, the probe will deliver 60% of the maximum power which the machine is able to produce

Programmable modes

The maximum aspiration rate, vacuum and phaco power, as well as the bottle height, can all be set using the VDU or keypad control.

Surgeons almost always have *pre-programmed combinations of settings* that they use for the different stages of phacoemulsification surgery. These are typically identified as 'Phaco 1', 'Phaco 2' etc when communicating with the assisting nurse. Since the combinations are stored in the software's memory, the machine's automated voice prompts often refer to them as 'Memory 1', 'Memory 2', etc. A unique combination of settings is also used for I/A.

In practice you will most likely start operating using your supervisor's preferred combinations of settings.

Phaco 1/Memory 1

This usually refers to the settings used for sculpting the grooves in the nucleus (see chapter 8). Significant vacuum is not required during this stage. Typical Phaco 1 settings are:

Max aspiration rate:	20cc/min
Max vacuum:	66mmHg*
Max phaco power:	60%
Bottle height:	65-105cm

* This is the lowest possible vacuum on our machine.

Phaco 2/Memory 2

This usually refers to settings used for emulsification of the four quadrants (chapter 8). Here vacuum is required to obtain a grip on lens fragments. Typical Phaco 2 settings are:

Max aspiration rate:	20cc/min
Max vacuum:	250mmHg
Max phaco power:	60%
Bottle height:	65-105cm

I/A

Since phaco power is not used during I/A (chapter 9 & 10), when you request I/A mode the footpedal control will change such that there will only be Positions 1 & 2, which function as previously. There is no longer a Position 3. Typical I/A settings are:

Max aspiration rate: 25cc/min
Max vacuum: 500mmHg
Bottle height: 65-105cm

Adapting settings

Settings can be changed for specific purposes. For example:

- phaco power may be increased in the case of a hard nucleus

- vacuum may be increased if you experience difficulty in getting a good grip on lens matter

(Until you are fairly experienced, such changes will usually be made at the direction of your supervisor when necessary.)

When making changes it is important always to remember the relationship between irrigation and aspiration

> → *the rate of irrigation must be sufficient to match the rate of aspiration.* If this is not the case (for example if the bottle height is low and the rate of aspiration relatively high), the anterior chamber will collapse

Influencing AC depth

Sometimes you may find that surgery is difficult because the anterior chamber is too deep or too shallow. In the absence of identifiable causes, manipulating settings may make operating easier:

AC too shallow

Raising the bottle height without altering the aspiration rate will tend to deepen the AC (the irrigation pressure is increased).

AC too deep

Lowering the bottle height without altering the aspiration rate may shallow the AC. Take care not to lower the bottle too much, which may result in collapse of the AC.

Pulsed phaco

During phacoemulsification, the jackhammer effect of the phaco needle tends to push lens matter away from the tip. Aspiration then draws the lens matter back onto the tip, only for it to be pushed away again. Because the needle oscillates continuously, some energy is delivered while the lens matter is not in contact with the tip, resulting in inefficiency.

In pulsed phaco, the phaco power is generated in *regular, repetitive short bursts, interrupted by brief microsecond pauses.* During the burst the lens matter is pushed away, and during the pause aspiration draws it back onto the tip. The result is that less energy is delivered while lens matter is not in contact with the tip

> → *energy is thus delivered more efficiently, and total energy expended in the eye may be reduced*

'Pulsed phaco mode' is selected by the assisting nurse using the VDU/keypad control. Once the mode is activated, engage Position 3 in the normal way to deliver pulsed energy.

Some surgeons use pulsed phaco routinely, usually during 'Phaco 2' (removal of the nuclear quadrants, chapter 10). Others request this mode in cases where they especially want to limit the total amount of energy used, for example in cases of hard nuclei or Fuch's corneal endothelial dystrophy.

Footnote
The controls to activate continuous irrigation and reflux may be different in your phaco machine. You should familiarise yourself with these.

8
Phacoemulsification

Two deep, perpendicular grooves which intersect at their midpoints are made in the lens. The appearance is thus of a cross (Fig 8.1). The nucleus is then cracked along these grooves, yielding four separate quadrants which are removed independently by emulsification with phaco power.

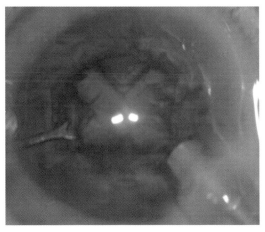

Fig 8.1 Two intersecting grooves made in the lens

sleeve. If necessary, twist the sleeve to adjust the amount of exposed tip.

Also ensure that the irrigation ports are directed sideways, as described previously.

Another instrument, usually referred to as the 'second intrument', is used to manipulate the lens and to protect the posterior capsule during phacoemulsification.

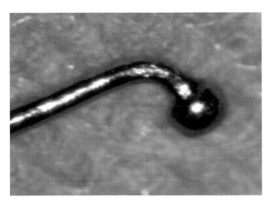

Fig 8.2 A mushroom (second instrument)

Instruments

The phaco equipment has been discussed. When the phaco probe is handed to you, check that the correct amount of needle tip is exposed beyond the end of the irrigation

Inserting the instruments

•   Before inserting the instruments, ensure that the patient's head position is correct (*with the iris perfectly in the horizontal plane*), as you should not make adjustments later when the instruments are in the eye.

- The phaco probe is held like a pen in your right hand, at an angle of about 30° with the horizontal (Fig 8.3). The *bevel of the tip faces downwards initially to aid passage through the section.*

- Position the phaco tip close to the corneal section and depress the footpedal into Position 1, activating irrigation.

- *With irrigation running*, advance the tip through the wound under microscopic vision and position it in the centre of the AC (depressing the bottom lip of the wound gently with the face of the bevel allows the point of the needle to pass cleanly under the upper lip).

- Holding the phaco probe in position, use your second hand to help you rotate it through 180°, so that the *bevel of the tip now faces upwards.*

- Without looking away from the microscope, accept the second instrument in your left hand.

- Insert the tip of the second instrument through the paracentesis and position it in the AC. To allow easy passage of the instrument through the paracentesis, ensure that its trajectory is the same as the plane of the wound i.e the

instrument must not be angled too steeply or too flat

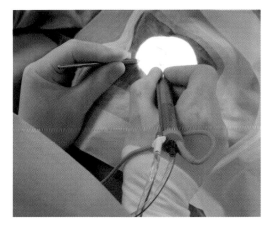

Fig 8.3 Correct handling of the instruments

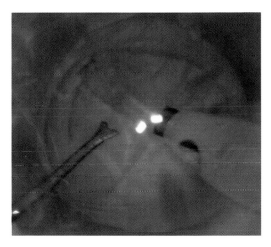

Fig 8.4 Correct initial positioning of the instruments in the AC

Note: *Irrigation must always be running when the phaco probe is in the eye*

→ if adjusting the microscope with your left foot, concentrate on not allowing the right pedal to come out of Position 1, so that irrigation is never interrupted

Place the eye in the primary position

During phacoemulsification it is essential to have the eye in the primary position (i.e. looking straight ahead with the iris in the horizontal plane) at all times. This ensures an optimal view against the best possible red reflex. This is particularly important when it comes to assessing the depth and extent of the grooves you are about to make.

Fig 8.5 shows the eye deviated out of the primary position. Notice how poor the view is compared with the same eye in Fig 8.1.

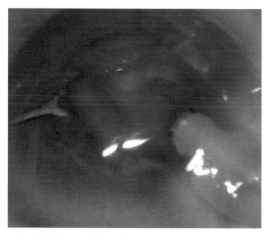

Fig 8.5 Poor view due to deviation out of the primary position

You may find after inserting the instruments that you have pushed the eye into depression by inadvertently lifting against the roof of the corneal section. If so, push gently down on the floor of the section with the phaco probe to return the eye to the correct position.

Appreciate that no matter where the eye is deviated, you can use the two instruments in combination to return it to the primary position and maintain it there.

Aspirate viscoelastic & loose cortex

So far you have kept the footpedal in Position 1 (irrigation only).

- Now depress the footpedal into Position 2 to aspirate the viscoelastic filling the AC *(footnote)*

  → move the phaco tip briefly around the AC while aspirating, without touching any structures. Ensure all the viscoelastic is removed (although viscoelastic is essentially transparent, you are able to see it, so you will know when you have removed it all)

You may find that, as a result of your hydrodissection with/without hydrodelamination, some of the anterior cortex has been disrupted

  → 'strands' of cortex may be seen to flay in the AC with the circulation of fluid; in some cases this loose cortex can obscure your view of the anterior lens surface

- Aspirate these strands by engaging them with the phaco tip with the footpedal in Position 2

→ this improves your view of the surface of the lens before you begin sculpting the grooves

→ you may increase the aspiration rate if necessary, by depressing the footpedal further within Position 2, in order to aspirate this cortex. However, do not use any phaco power yet

The first groove

- Position the phaco tip overlying the lens cortex, just in front of the capsulorhexis at the 11 o'clock position (i.e. in front of the sub-incisional rhexis)

  → the distance from the capsulorhexis that you commence the groove will depend on the size of the rhexis. For a small capsulorhexis you will need to start closer to the capsule margin

- Depress the footpedal into Position 3, activating phaco power

  → *do not be tentative in this step*, trying just to edge the pedal into Position 3; rather depress it confidently a few centimetres into Position 3 to generate a continual burst of phaco power

→ however, you will *not* need to depress the pedal maximally at this stage

- At the same time as activating phaco power, in a single movement:

  → advance the phaco tip deeper so that it penetrates the lens to a depth of about $1/2$ of the length of the exposed needle tip

  → simultaneously advance it towards the rhexis on the opposite side, stopping short of the rhexis margin

  → maintain a constant depth

The result will be a groove in the lens.

- *Deactivate phaco power* by returning the footpedal to Position 1 *while you move the phaco tip back to the original start position.*

- Deepen the groove by repeating the above steps until it is about as deep as the length of the exposed tip.

- In order for the groove to be deepened further, it has to be widened to accommodate the irrigation sleeve. The width of the groove needs to be about $1\frac{1}{2}$ times the diameter of the phaco tip

  → use grooving strokes to remove an equal sliver from each of the side walls of the groove to achieve the desired width (Fig 8.6)

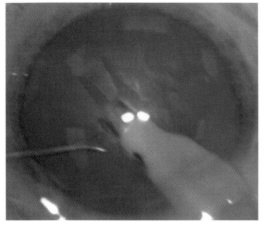

Fig 8.6 Widening the groove by removing a sliver of side wall

Principles guiding further deepening of the groove

The lens is thickest in the centre. In order for you to be able to crack the nucleus into quadrants, grooves need to be *deep centrally rather than peripherally*. Fig 8.7 illustrates the following:

→ a groove that extends deep peripherally will not weaken the nucleus sufficiently in the centre for it to crack

→ a groove that extends deep peripherally brings the phaco tip dangerously close to the posterior capsule, which may be inadvertently damaged

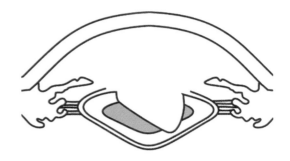

Fig 8.7 INCORRECTLY constructed groove going deep peripherally

There is a natural tendency to direct the phaco tip deeper as you come towards the end of a grooving stroke. This must be resisted as it will lead to the type of groove shown in Fig 8.7.

Therefore:

• Consider the natural cross-sectional contour of the posterior capsule as you now make additional strokes to deepen the groove further

→ you should no longer maintain a constant depth with these grooving strokes: instead, aim to make the groove deepest in the centre of the lens (*because the probe passes through the corneal section and over the sub-incisional rhexis, in practice this means that maximal depth should be attained soon after beginning the grooving stroke*)

→ as the stroke continues peripherally, you should direct the tip shallower. This keeps it a safe distance away from the posterior capsule, as shown in Fig 8.8. The base of your groove should thus follow the contour of the posterior capsule

under the anterior capsule) carries an increased risk of damage to both anterior and posterior capsule.

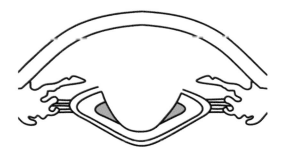

Fig 8.8 Correct groove contour – deep centrally, shallower peripherally

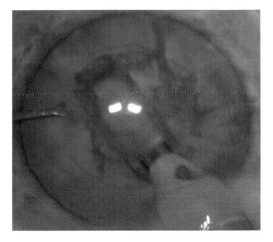

Fig 8.9 First groove

At this stage the groove does NOT need to be deepened to the point where you think you would be able to crack the nucleus. It only needs to be sufficiently deep to allow for the next step, which is rotation of the lens

> → your supervisor should advise you when the depth is sufficient for rotation, but as a guide a central depth of about twice the length of the exposed phaco tip should suffice

Extent of the groove

With an average sized rhexis the groove *does not need to extend more peripherally than the margin of the capsulorhexis* (Fig 8.1). Applying phaco peripheral to this (i.e.

Rotation of the lens

You must now rotate the lens through 90° so that a second groove can be formed perpendicular to the first. In order to rotate the lens anti-clockwise, position the instruments as shown in Fig 8.10

> → the tip of the second instrument is inserted deeply into the distal part of the groove and exerts a force on the left lateral wall

> → the phaco tip is inserted deeply into the proximal part of the groove and exerts a force on the right lateral wall

• Use both instruments simultaneously to apply a rotational force.

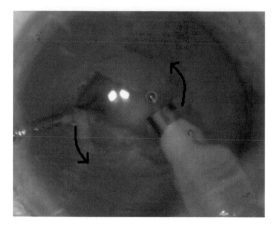

Fig 8.10 Rotation of the lens

Key points to appreciate are:

- the instruments must be inserted deeply into the groove in order to have sufficient grip on the lens matter. However, take care only to exert horizontal/rotational forces on the side walls of the groove – *do not push down on the lens*

- the ease with which the lens rotates *is highly dependant on your hydrodissection/hydrodelamination* performed earlier

Difficulty with lens rotation

You may find that the lens will not rotate. Trying to exert excessive force may:

i) cause the instruments to tear through the lens matter, disrupting the architecture of your groove and making things much more difficult. This happens especially in the case of a soft nucleus

ii) displace the lens and capsule together as a complex, *placing stress on the zonules* which will rupture if too much force is applied

If the lens will not rotate:

→ ensure that your groove is deep enough to allow adequate grip for the instruments

→ ensure that the instrument tips are placed deeply within the grooves for the same reason

→ ensure that you are exerting a purely rotational force against the side walls of the groove, without pushing downwards

→ attempting to rotate the lens the other way (clockwise) may prove successful

→ *have a low threshold for performing further hydrodissection early*. Doing this earlier rather than later may prevent damage to the groove architecture and/or zonules through attempted forced rotation. Remove both instruments and perform further hydrodissection at various sites as described in chapter 6

The second groove

Once the lens has been rotated though 90°, you will note that the first groove is not symmetrical about the midpoint of the lens (Fig 8.11). The second groove:

> → must be perpendicular to the first

> → *must pass through the centre of the lens, NOT the midpoint of the groove already constructed*

- Commence the second groove as for the first, just in front of the sub-incisional rhexis margin. Extend it across the first groove towards the opposite rhexis, stopping short of the margin.

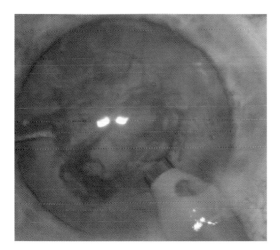

Fig 8.11 Commencement of the second groove

- Widen and then deepen it to the same depth as the first groove, ensuring again that maximal depth is obtained in the centre of the lens.

- You may find that the lens moves

slightly during grooving, making it difficult for you to keep the second groove aligned perpendicular to the first

> → it may be helpful to stabilize the lens by inserting the tip of the second instrument into the first groove while sculpting the second (Fig 8.12)

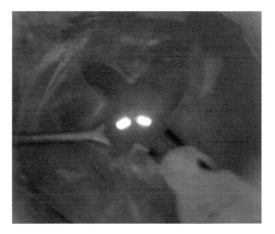

Fig 8.12 Stabilizing the lens with the second instrument positioned in the first groove

Further rotation and grooving

- Rotate the lens through a further 90° using the instruments as before. The first groove has thus been rotated through 180° and is once again perpendicular to the corneal section (Fig 8.13).

- You thus have easier access to what started as the proximal portion of the first groove and can now sculpt this so that the entire groove is symmetrical about its midpoint.

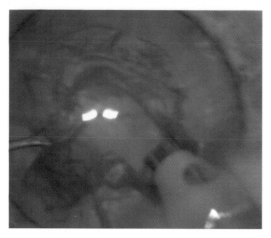

Fig 8.13 The original groove has been rotated through 180°

- Rotating another 90° allows you to do the same for the second groove.

Deepening the grooves

The lens must be sufficiently thinned by the grooves to allow cracking into four quadrants. However, *the danger of grooving too deeply is a full thickness groove through the entire lens with damage to the posterior capsule.*

An appreciation of what depth is required must be gained by experience, with instruction from your supervisor.

However, the following points should prove helpful:

- *Always keep the eye in the primary position.* This ensures that the grooves lie perfectly in the horizontal plane and are well silhouetted against a good red reflex. Correction of incorrect eye posi-

tion can cause a marked improvement in your view and in your ability to perceive the relative depth of structures. (cf Fig. 8.1 & 8.5).

Note
When first learning phacoemulsification, you will find that you have so much to think about at this stage of the operation that it is easy to let the eye drift out of the primary position without realising it. Your view deteriorates as a result and you may find yourself struggling without knowing why

→ *it is useful to get into the habit of **regularly checking that the eye is in the primary position** and correcting things if necessary*

- Remember to adjust the focus downwards as the groove deepens, so that the base of the groove stays in focus.

- Your depth of field increases as magnification decreases. Alternatively, high magnification allows better visualisation of the fine architecture of the groove bases

→ if you are having difficulty gauging your depth, try changing the magnification – zooming in or out may make things clearer

- During sculpting it is *better to take too little than too much* (another sculpting stroke is far preferable to a VR referral!) Using small increments is prudent, especially when first learning.

- Classically the red reflex is said to become brighter in the groove as the posterior plate (base of the groove) is progressively thinned

    → however, the helpfulness of this sign will depend on the density of the cataract. An early cataract will allow a bright red reflex even before the lens is significantly thinned in the grooves, while in the case of a very dense cataract you may be very close to the posterior capsule before the reflex brightens appreciably

- When learning, there is a tendency to apply phaco power tentatively/gently by edging the footpedal only slightly into Position 3. This may yield insufficient energy (especially in the case of a hard nucleus), so that instead of emulsifying/grooving the nucleus, the phaco tip simply pushes it. In this case the groove does not progress as expected, and you may find that you either push the nucleus out of correct alignment or push it away from you with the phaco tip

    → be sure to apply sufficient phaco power by *depressing the pedal well into Position 3* and observing the reaction at the phaco tip. Depress the pedal further if there is not adequate emulsification at the tip. In the case of a dense nucleus you may need to depress the pedal

fully, or even increase the power setting (chapter 7)

- Remember to concentrate on making the groove deep centrally, as opposed to peripherally.

The finished result after completing the grooves is shown in Fig 8.1

Cracking the nucleus into quadrants

- Examine the proximal and distal parts of each groove to determine where the nucleus appears easiest to crack

    → determine where the posterior plate appears to be thinnest; and/or

    → determine where the groove architecture would allow the best grip for your instruments (see below)

- Align your chosen groove so that it runs perpendicular to the corneal section, with the targeted area opposite the section at the 5 o'clock position.

- Insert the phaco tip and the tip of the second instrument *deeply into the base of the groove* at its distal end (Fig 8.14), *without pressing down on the lens.*

- Gently use the phaco tip to exert a horizontal force against the side wall of the groove in the direction shown in the figure. Simultaneously use the second instrument to exert a similar force against the other side wall in the opposite direction

→ these forces should be *purely horizontal* – do not push downwards on the lens

→ in this manoeuvre the phaco probe should pivot on an imaginary point in the corneal section. Similarly the second instrument pivots on a point in the paracentesis. Thus no stress should be placed on the margins of these wounds

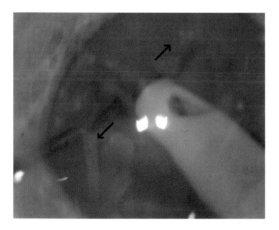

Fig 8.14 Positioning and movement of the instruments to crack the nucleus

→ this manoeuvre will result in a crack appearing in the base of the groove, starting peripherally and extending towards the centre. The two fragments are seen to separate, with bright-

ening of the red reflex in the crack

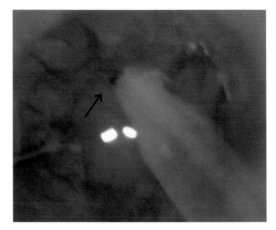

Fig 8.15 Brightening of the red reflex in the crack

→ the tips of the instruments should be separated sufficiently so that the crack extends to the midpoint of the groove

→ it is not necessary for the crack to extend the full length of the groove. Therefore *do not splay your instruments excessively* in an attempt to achieve this – doing so may place stress on the capsule

• Rotate the lens either way through 90° and repeat the step in the next distal groove. A second crack results.

• Rotating a further 90° in the same direction brings the first groove into alignment again. Repeating the manoeuvre should result in the first crack now extending the full length of this groove.

- Rotating another 90° and repeating the step once more should lead to the second crack also now extending the full length of its groove

  → the result is that the nucleus is now split into four separate quadrants

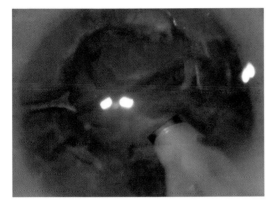

Fig 8.16 Intersecting cracks seen in the bases of the grooves. The nucleus has been cracked into four separate quadrants

Difficulty cracking

- The most common cause for difficulty in cracking the nucleus is *inadequate depth of the grooves, especially in the centre.*

  The temptation is to extend the grooves peripherally, but this will usually be less helpful than further deepening centrally, and may endanger the posterior capsule.

  You will need to re-examine the grooves carefully to see where further thinning of the posterior plate is possible, employing the principles outlined above.

- Another possibility is that you may not have optimal grip on the lens matter with the instruments

  → both tips need to be inserted into the *depth* of the distal groove. Failure to achieve this positioning may lead to pieces of the side walls breaking off as the instruments are separated, destroying the architecture of the groove

Hard nucleus
In the case of a hard nucleus, it is often useful to cross the instruments and exert the forces as shown in Fig 8.17.

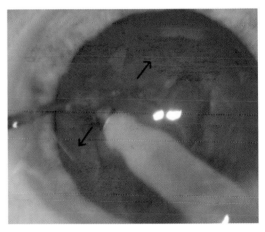

Fig 8.17 Crossing the instruments when cracking

Phaco of the quadrants

The nucleus is now emulsified one quadrant at a time. Emulsification of the quadrants is performed with different phaco settings to those used for groove formation (chapter 7). Therefore ask the assisting nurse for 'Phaco 2'. The change of settings is confirmed with an audio prompt from the machine before proceeding.

The 'safe zone'

We use this term to refer to an area where you should aim to have your phaco tip most of the time during the remainder of phaco. The zone is a *small area centered around the centre of the pupil, in the plane of the anterior capsule*.

It is thus a safe distance from the

- posterior capsule

- capsulorhexis margin

- corneal endothelium

Inadvertently touching any structure with the vibrating phaco tip will cause damage – hence the importance of a safe zone in which to work.

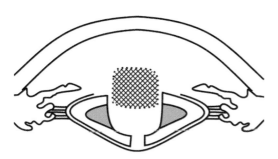

Fig 8.18 The 'safe zone'

The first quadrant

Each quadrant must be unlocked/disengaged from its adjacent quadrants and moved into the safe zone before it can be emulsified. The first quadrant is the most difficult to unlock from the rest

→ therefore identify the quadrant which is bordered by the best cracks i.e. the one you feel will be most likely to disengage

- Rotate the lens so that the apex of this quadrant is opposite the corneal section at the 5 o'clock position (Fig 8.20).

- Activate aspiration by depressing the pedal into Position 2.

- Advance the phaco tip carefully towards point X shown in Fig 8.19. This lies on the apical surface of the quadrant and is a safe distance from the anterior and posterior capsule

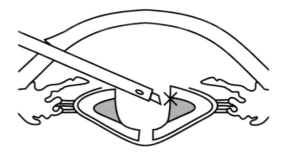

Fig 8.19 Point to target with the phaco tip

→ as the phaco tip touches the surface of the quadrant, it will begin to occlude. The pitch of the machine's sound output will rise as vacuum is generated

- When the tip is fully occluded and the sound output indicates good vacuum,

you should have an adequate 'grip' on the lens matter. Maintain the footpedal position and withdraw the tip towards the safe zone

→ if the cracks are adequate and sufficient vacuum is maintained, the quadrant should stay adherent to the phaco tip, unlock from its adjacent quadrants, and be drawn towards the safe zone

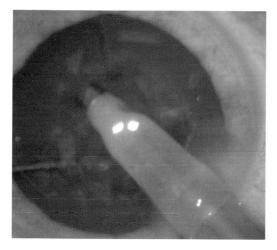

Fig 8.20 Unlocking a quadrant in order to draw it towards the safe zone

• However, it sometimes happens that the tip pulls away from the targeted quadrant without disengaging it. In this case, repeat the above sequence as necessary, using progressively higher aspiration rates to achieve higher vacuum and a better grip on the lens matter.

If this is still unsuccessful, try the following manoeuvre:

• Proceed initially as above. As the phaco tip touches the quadrant and vacuum starts to be generated, *simultaneously*

→ *gently edge the footpedal just a little into Position 3* and then return to Position 2, resulting in a short burst of *weak* phaco

→ advance the tip about a millimetre into the substance of the fragment

With the tip now embedded in the substance of the quadrant there should be better occlusion, generating more vacuum and hence better grip.

• Maintaining vacuum, withdraw the tip towards the safe zone – the quadrant should disengage.

Difficulty disengaging the first quadrant

Sometimes you may find that as you withdraw the phaco tip after engaging the quadrant, a fragment breaks off, leaving the bulk of the quadrant behind. This implies that you have a good grip on the quadrant, but that it has not been adequately separated from the adjacent quadrants to allow it to unlock.

If you experience difficulty disengaging the selected quadrant, consider targeting one of the others. If none of the quadrants brings success you will need to re-examine the cracks.

- Place the tips of both instruments into each of the grooves bordering a quadrant in turn. Employing the usual cracking action, make sure that the selected quadrant is fully separated from its adjacent quadrants by *complete* cracks.

A useful tip

Sometimes you may find that on trying to draw a quadrant towards the safe zone, one of its adjacent quadrants is pulled centrally also. This implies that you have a good grip on the quadrant, but that it has not been properly cracked from the adjacent quadrant which also moves. The fact that the adjacent quadrant moves with it prevents the targeted quadrant from unlocking.

Re-cracking is one option, but you may also try the following:

- Use the second instrument to press

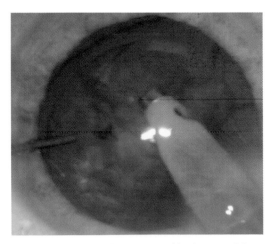

Fig 8.21 Using the second instrument to hold back an adjacent quadrant while drawing the targeted quadrant to the safe zone

gently against the apical surface of the adjacent quadrant while you attempt to disengage the targeted quadrant, as illustrated in Fig 8.21. This prevents the adjacent quadrant from moving and may help to unlock the fragment.

Safe zone phaco

Once you have unlocked the first quadrant and drawn it into the safe zone, you can begin to emulsify it with phaco power. The principles are as follows:

- *Do not apply phaco power unless there is lens matter against the phaco-tip (footnote)*

  → in the case of a large fragment it must be engaged with vacuum before phaco is applied

  → later, when only small fragments remain, they will not occlude the tip to generate vacuum, so you should see these fragments sucked up against the tip before applying phaco

- Phaco power is applied in *bursts*, usually lasting a second or so. The phaco causes the nuclear matter to disintegrate into smaller fragments. After a burst of phaco, return to Position 2 and reassess the situation. Get a grip on a new sizeable fragment and then deliver the next burst of phaco

  → *emulsification is thus per-*

formed with brief applications of phaco power, interrupted by pauses in which you observe the effect and decide on the next area of lens matter to target

)   *do not simply apply continuous phaco power until the whole quadrant has been emulsified*: doing this results in a significant proportion of the energy being delivered when no lens matter is in contact with the phaco tip, which is inefficient

→   in addition, the pauses interrupting the phaco power allow for cooling of the phaco needle, reducing the chance of causing a phaco burn

- *Keep the phaco tip in the safe zone at all times while applying phaco-power.* As the quadrant is emulsified, the fragments that result will move within the AC and may drift out of the safe zone

→   do not chase after a fragment outside the safe zone while applying phaco power. Rather return to Position 2 and move the tip to the fragment. Once you have a grip on the fragment, move it back to the safe zone before applying phaco power

- *Avoid 'bayoneting' fragments*: With large fragments the temptation is to phaco all the way through the lens matter. However, since you will not be able to see what lies immediately behind a large fragment, this is unsafe

→   rather phaco $^2/_3$ of the way into the fragment, return to Position 1, disengage it with the help of your second instrument, and then target a new area

Use of the second instrument

The second instrument has the following uses at this stage:

- It can be used to **manipulate lens matter**, pushing/pulling a targeted fragment towards the phaco tip. It can be used to disengage lens matter from the tip, for example after phaco'ing partially through a large fragment.

- It is also used to *protect the posterior capsule from the phaco tip*. For this purpose the tip of the second instrument must be positioned deep to the fragment being phaco'd → therefore just deep to the safe zone. This prevents the possibility of forwards movement of the posterior capsule into the safe zone

→   do not push any structures downwards with the second instrument. Simply *interposition* the tip between the safe zone and the posterior capsule (Fig 8.21 & 8.24)

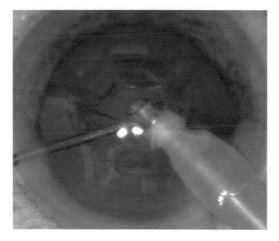

Fig 8.21 Emulsifying lens matter in the safe zone with the second instrument positioned deep to this

This use of the second instrument becomes more important as more quadrants are removed, because there is less lens matter left in the capsular bag to prevent forwards movement of the posterior capsule.

Note
Take care not to touch the tips of the two instruments together while applying phaco power → this can lead to shedding of metal fragments in the eye.

The remaining quadrants

After the first quadrant has been completely emulsified, select the next quadrant which you deem most likely to separate from the others.

- Rotate the remaining quadrants until the apex of the selected quadrant is opposite the corneal section, at the 5

o'clock position

→ it is often helpful to push against the free side wall of one of the end quadrants with the tip of the second instrument (Fig 8.22) to aid rotation at this stage

- Engage the selected quadrant and draw it to the safe zone to be phaco'd as for the previous quadrant.

- Repeat for the third quadrant.

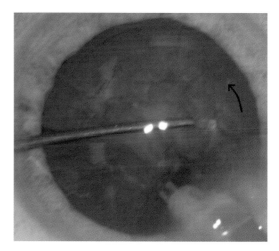

Fig 8.22 Pushing against a free side wall to aid rotation (2 quadrants remaining)

The last quadrant

The last quadrant merits special attention, because once it has been drawn to the safe zone there are no more quadrants left in the capsular bag to prevent forwards movement of the posterior capsule

→ *thus the second instrument*

must be held deep to the last quadrant while phaco is being applied at this stage. If you need to manipulate a fragment, first stop applying phaco power before manipulating it. Then reposition the second instrument deep to the fragment before continuing phaco

Removing the instruments

After all the nuclear lens matter has been removed, return the footpedal to Position 1. Then remove the second instrument, followed by the phaco probe, with irrigation still running

> → only the nucleus is intentionally removed at this stage – the epinucleus and cortex are left in the capsular bag (in practice some epinucleus and cortex are inevitably removed together with the nucleus, but you should not deliberately target any soft lens matter in this step of the operation)

Nucleus is differentiated by:

- its characteristic brown colour or tinge (depending on the amount of nuclear sclerosis present)

- its hard consistency in comparison with epinucleus and cortex

Potential pitfalls

Many potential pitfalls have already been addressed in this chapter. Additional points follow:

Stop sooner rather than later
If at any point something doesn't look quite right/you feel that you are not in control → STOP.

More damage is done if you continue in spite of a complication, for example a posterior capsule tear. Your view may be better than your supervisor's – if you suspect something is wrong, ask him/her to have a closer look. Do not rely on your supervisor to detect complications.

Supervisors are reassured when they know they can trust you to stop if you are unsure.

Losing your view
If your view deteriorates it is likely that you have moved the eye out of the primary position

> → avoid exerting unnecessary forces with the instruments, which will deviate the eye; for example, inadvertently lifting against the roof of the corneal section with the phaco probe will push the eye into depression

> → use the instruments to apply corrective forces; for example, pushing down on the floor of

the section will return an eye in depression to the primary position

→ ensure that the patient has not moved his/her head; if necessary remove the instruments from the eye and reposition the head correctly

Corneal stress lines

If the phaco probe is not orientated radially, stress lines in the cornea may result, obscuring your view. The probe should always pass perpendicular to the section, directed towards/through the centre of the pupil. Therefore, use the second instrument to move targeted lens matter to the 5 o'clock position opposite the corneal section before engaging it with the phaco tip, rather than angle the phaco probe to engage it at other positions (Fig 8.23).

Failure to protect the posterior capsule

If there is insufficient lens matter splinting it in place, the posterior capsule may move forwards. Only part of the capsule may billow forwards if one/a few quadrants have been removed, or the whole capsule may move forwards if there are no quadrants left in the bag.

To prevent capsular damage with the phaco tip, it is safe practice to keep the tip of the second instrument deep to the lens matter you are emulsifying at all times.

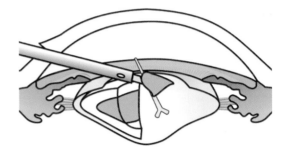

Fig 8.24 Correctly positioned second instrument prevents the possibility of the posterior capsule billowing forwards into the safe zone

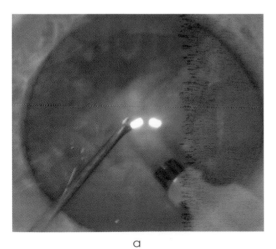

a

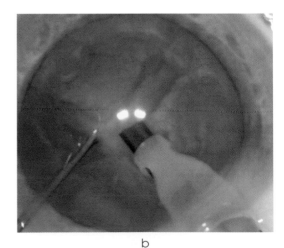

b

Fig 8.23 (a) 2 quadrants have been removed; (b) one of the remaining quadrants is moved to the 5 o'clock position before being engaged

PHACO FUNDAMENTALS – A GUIDE FOR TRAINEE OPHTHALMIC SURGEONS

Phaco burn

A phaco burn results if heat generated by the vibrating phaco needle burns the margins of the corneal wound. It is recognised by white discolouration of the cornea around the section. The result is a wound which is unlikely to self-seal and which will be slow to heal. To minimise the chances of a burn:

- aspirate all the viscoelastic from the AC before commencing phaco[1]

- be efficient in your use of phaco power, only applying it when lens matter is up against the phaco tip[2]

- *avoid pressing too firmly against the wound margins with the probe* → this compresses the irrigation sleeve and compromises cooling at that site

Shallow AC

A shallow anterior chamber makes things difficult because there is not much space for you to manoeuvre the instruments comfortably. If you find that the AC is shallower than expected, exclude the following reversible causes:

- check for excessive leakage of BSS around your second instrument or phaco probe during irrigation

    → leakage around your second instrument implies that you are pushing down on the floor or lifting up against the roof of the paracentesis; allow the instrument to pivot in the wound, without distorting it

    → it may be necessary to place a suture at a lateral aspect of the section to tighten the seal of the section around the phaco probe

- a Valsalva effect can cause shallowing of the AC → ensure that the patient is not holding his/her breath

- with certain palpebral apertures, the lids and speculum combine to form a ring which exerts pressure on the posterior segment, causing shallowing of the AC

    → lifting the speculum forwards slightly may relieve this effect and deepen the AC

Note

If the AC shallows rapidly during the operation, you must *consider and exclude a suprachoroidal haemorrhage*. Signs of this complication include:

- shallow AC
- hard eye
- darkening of the red reflex
- tendency for the iris to prolapse through the section

    → if this is suspected your supervisor will need to manage further

If all of the above have been excluded, raising the bottle height (chapter 7) may result in deepening of the AC.

Footnotes

1. Viscoelastic moves more slowly through the aspiration duct than BSS, so it may limit flow through the irrigation/aspiration system, reducing cooling. If you apply phaco power before all the viscoelastic has been removed from the AC, you increase the risk of causing a phaco burn.

2. Applying phaco power while waiting for lens matter to come up against the tip is an inefficient use of energy. Realise that the more phaco energy you expend, the more likely you are to encounter complications such as phaco burns.

9

Removal of the Epinucleus

After removal of the nuclear quadrants, there will be residual lens matter left in the capsular bag. This will always comprise some cortex, the removal of which is described in the next chapter. However, if you achieved a thorough hydrodelamination, there will also be a significant amount of epinucleus which you will need to remove.

Identifying epinucleus

In terms of its characteristics, it is helpful to think of epinucleus as lying somewhere between nucleus and cortex. Your supervisor should help you to distinguish these types of lens matter. The following points should prove helpful:

Consistency
Epinucleus is softer than nucleus, but harder than cortex. These types of lens matter therefore *behave differently* when they are engaged by an instrument or when BSS circulates through the AC

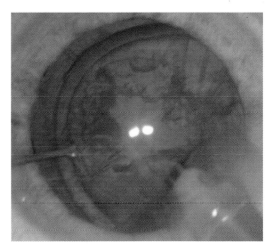

Fig 9.1 A 'bowl' of epinucleus remaining after nucleus removal

→ nuclear lens matter is not easily deformable and usually requires emulsification with phaco power before it can be aspirated

→ epinucleus does not require emulsification to be aspirated, but is less deformable than cortex. It thus provides more resistance to aspiration than cortex does

→ cortex is easily deformable and so passes readily through the I/A aspiration port once it has been freed from the capsule (chapter 10)

Location

Cortex is the most peripheral lens matter in the capsular bag - it lies up against the capsule. The nucleus forms the centre of the lens. Epinucleus is situated between cortex and the nucleus.

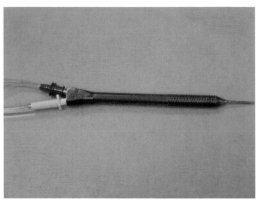

Fig 9.3 Straight I/A handpiece

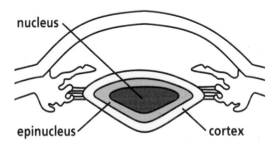

Fig 9.2 The lens in cross section

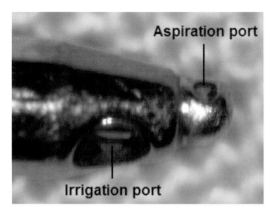

Fig 9.4 Straight I/A tip

Colour

Epinucleus and cortex lack the characteristic brownish colour that the nucleus has when nuclear sclerosis is present.

Instruments

Straight I/A: (I/A = irrigation/aspiration) *The safest way to remove epinucleus is to use the straight I/A handpiece.* This has two irrigation ports and an aspiration port.

• As with the phaco handpiece, irrigation is gravity fed and is activated by depressing the footpedal into Position

1. The rate of irrigation does *not* alter if the footpedal is depressed further within Position 1.

• Aspiration is activated by engaging Position 2 with the footpedal (irrigation continues to run). This is signalled by a constant sound output from the phaco machine. Higher rates of aspiration are generated by depressing the pedal further (as when using the phaco probe)

→ if the I/A aspiration port is

occluded by lens matter while you aspirate, vacuum is generated (in the case of a peristaltic machine). Increasing the aspiration rate generates higher vacuum. The increase in vacuum is signalled by a rise in pitch of the sound output

I/A mode

I/A mode refers to the programmable machine settings that apply when using this instrument. As with the phaco modes, values can be pre-programmed to suit your preferences. You can also adjust the settings intra-operatively while performing I/A.

Typical values are:

Max aspiration rate: 25cc/min
Max vacuum: 500mmHg
Bottle height: 65-105cm

The I/A handpiece does not deliver phaco power, so the footpedal does not have Position 3 when I/A mode is operational.

Second instrument

The second instrument is the same as that used during phacoemulsification (Fig 8.2).

Method

- Ask the assisting nurse to select 'I/A mode' – the machine will give audio confirmation.

- Accept the straight I/A probe in your right hand. This is held like a pen, as for the phaco probe. The aspiration port must face upwards.

- Position the I/A tip close to the corneal section and engage Position 1 with the pedal, activating irrigation.

- With irrigation running, insert the probe via the corneal section. Depressing the floor of the corneal wound gently with the tip aids its smooth passage under the roof of the section into the AC (Fig 9.5).

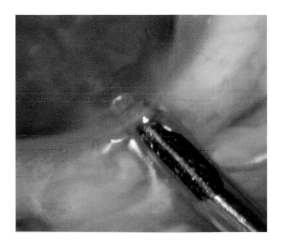

Fig 9.5 Inserting the I/A probe into the AC

- Position the I/A tip in the safe zone

  → *irrigation must always be running when you have the I/A probe inserted*

  → *keep the aspiration port directed upwards and in view at all times*

- Accept the second instrument in your left hand and insert it into the AC via the paracentesis.

- Position the tip of the second instrument *just deep to the safe zone,* in the centre of the AC (Fig 9.6)

    → take care not to press down on the underlying lens matter or posterior capsule

- Still irrigating only, advance the I/A tip towards the epinucleus situated at the 5 o'clock position, opposite the corneal section

    → the I/A probe thus passes over the tip of your second instrument

    → keep a safe distance away from the capsulorhexis margin

- When the I/A tip reaches the epinucleus, activate aspiration. *Use a low rate initially*

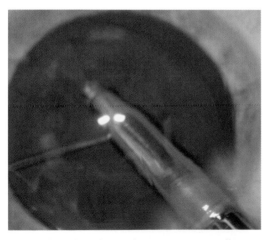

Fig 9.6 The I/A probe passes over the second instrument as you advance it towards the epinucleus at 5 o'clock

- → you may see epinucleus become engaged in the aspiration port

    → if not, try a slightly higher aspiration rate

- The epinucleus will occlude the port and you will hear the pitch of the audio output rise as vacuum is generated, giving you a 'grip' on the epinucleus

    → once the port is occluded and vacuum has been generated, *maintain aspiration but do not attempt to aspirate the epinucleus by increasing the rate yet*

- With epinucleus engaged, withdraw the I/A tip back to the safe zone

    → if you lose grip on the lens matter, try again with a higher aspiration rate

- Notice how the epinucleus is now wrapped around the tip of the second instrument, as shown in Fig 9.7 & 9.8.

- Now use the following manoeuvre to *free the epinucleus in the subincisional region*:

    → move the tip of the second instrument a few millimetres towards the 5 o'clock position and then back again (double headed arrow, Fig 9.8)

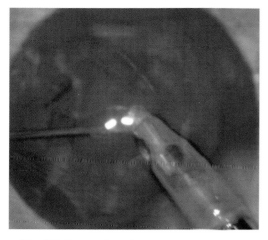

Fig 9.7 Epinucleus has been engaged and drawn to the safe zone. The 'bowl' of epinucleus is now wrapped around the second instrument

→ because the epinucleus is wrapped around the tip, this action pulls the subincisional epinucleus towards 5 o'clock (single headed arrow, Fig 9.8)

• Repeat this a few times as necessary, progressively dislodging the epinucleus from the subincisional area.

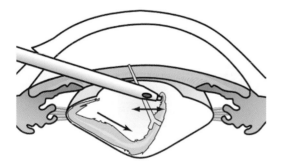

Fig 9.8 Epinucleus is wrapped around the second instrument; moving the second instrument dislodges the subincisional epinucleus

• As the subincisional epinucleus is freed, increase the aspiration rate to aspirate lens matter engaged at the I/A tip

→ because epinucleus is denser than cortex (for which the I/A probe is routinely used, see chapter 10), you may need to use comparatively high aspiration rates here. You may need to depress the footpedal maximally, or even adjust the machine settings to allow higher vacuum (chapter 7)

→ note that the ***epinucleus is thus aspirated around the tip of the second instrument***, as shown in Fig 9.9

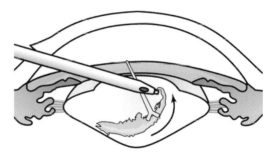

Fig 9.9 Epinucleus is aspirated around the second instrument

→ using the above technique, the 'bowl' of epinucleus tends to be freed as an intact structure which you systematically aspirate in the safe zone. Usually the lens matter does not fragment into separate pieces

(If you do not use the above technique to free the subincisional epinucleus first, but simply draw epinucleus from the 5 o'clock position to the safe zone and then increase aspiration, the 'bowl' may fragment. You may be left with epinucleus in the subincisional region only, which then becomes more difficult to deal with.)

If there are any residual pieces of epinucleus after the above manoeuvre, proceed as follows:

- Position the second instrument tip just deep to the safe zone.

- With the pedal in Position 1, advance the I/A tip to the targeted lens matter.

- Activate aspiration to engage the epinucleus and draw it to the safe zone

    → increase the aspiration rate if necessary to maintain a hold on the lens matter

- Once in the safe zone, increase the aspiration rate as necessary to aspirate the epinucleus.

- If residual epinucleus remains subincisionally, it may be easier to use the 90° I/A, which is described in chapter 10.

- Once all the epinucleus has been aspirated, return to irrigation only and remove the second instrument from the AC. Proceed to remove the cortex as described in the next chapter.

Using the phaco probe to remove epinucleus

An alternative is to use the phaco probe to aspirate the epinucleus.

Advantage
Epinucleus is aspirated more readily through the phaco tip than the smaller I/A aspiration port. In cases where epinucleus is unusually hard, you may encounter difficulty aspirating it with the I/A probe. Using the phaco probe in such cases may be easier.

Disadvantage
Using the phaco probe may be more dangerous

→ because epinucleus can be aspirated very quickly by the phaco probe, movement of lens matter may be rapid and less controlled

→ the sharper edges of the phaco needle are more likely to damage the capsule if you inadvertently touch it

→ the I/A aspiration port can be orientated so that it faces upwards, away from the posterior capsule, and is visible at all times, whereas the phaco needle is directed towards the capsule

Method
This is similar to the method described for the straight I/A.

- Position the phaco tip in the safe zone,

and the second instrument tip just deep to this.

- Irrigating only, advance the phaco tip towards the epinucleus closest to the 5 o'clock position.

- *Keep a safe distance from the capsulorhexis margin and posterior capsule* → this is especially important if the epinucleus is positioned more peripherally in the capsular fornix.

- Now activate *low rate* aspiration, such that epinucleus becomes engaged at the phaco tip

    → initially your aim is only to engage the epinucleus, not to aspirate it. Because epinucleus is readily aspirated by the phaco probe, you need to use a low aspiration rate

- With epinucleus engaged, draw the phaco tip back to the safe zone. Increase aspiration to maintain a grip if necessary.

- Then proceed using a similar technique to that described for the I/A probe.

- Once all the epinucleus has been aspirated, return to irrigation only. With irrigation running, withdraw the second instrument and then the phaco probe from the AC.

Note
Phaco power is not required during this step

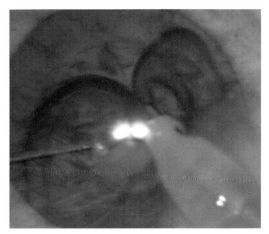

Fig 9.10 Epinucleus being aspirated around the second instrument with the phaco probe

Potential pitfalls

Capsular damage
The most important potential complication is damage to the capsule. To minimise the risk of this:

- use high rates of aspiration only when necessary and only in the safe zone

- always keep the tip of the second instrument deep to the I/A or phaco probe

- keep the I/A aspiration port directed upwards and in view

- if you choose to use the phaco probe, take special care *when initially engaging the epinucleus*

    → if you use a high aspiration rate at this point, you may inadvertently aspirate the epinucleus. *This can happen very quickly*, in which case you will suddenly find yourself aspirating close to the capsule, with no epinucleus left between the phaco tip and the capsule

- when using the second instrument in combination with the probe to dislodge the epinucleus from the subincisional region, use *repeated small movements* to minimise stress placed on the zonules

10

Irrigation/Aspiration (I/A)

Cortical lens matter, which remains in the capsular bag after removal of the nucleus and epinucleus, is removed by aspiration. This step is also referred to as cortical clearance.

Instruments

The straight I/A probe (Fig 9.3 & 9.4), which is described in the previous chapter, is used initially.

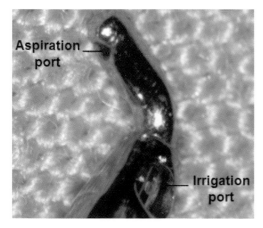

Fig 10.1 90° I/A

The 90° I/A probe (Fig 10.1) may be used to complete the removal of cortex. This instrument similarly has an aspiration port and two irrigation ports. The footpedal controls for the straight and 90° I/A probes are the same (chapters 7 and 9).

Surgical anatomy

Fig 10.2 illustrates that after removal of the nucleus and epinucleus, a layer of cortical lens matter remains against the capsule. This usually covers the posterior capsule and sweeps around the equatorial zone to extend under the anterior leaf of the capsule.

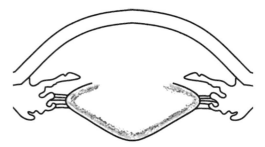

Fig 10.2 Cortex remains in the capsular bag after removal of the nucleus and epinucleus

In Fig 10.3 cortex is seen to extend under the anterior capsule, and in this case past the capsulorhexis margin. The wispy free ends of cortex typically flail about with the circulation of fluid in the AC.

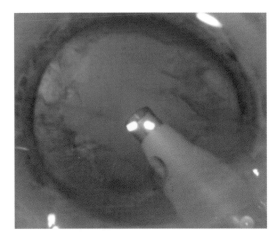

Fig 10.3 Cortex extends under the anterior capsule and past the rhexis margin

Method

- Begin by inspecting the anterior and posterior capsule to ensure there is no tear.

- Ask the assisting nurse to activate 'I/A mode' (chapter 7) – the machine will give an audible confirmation.

- Insert the straight I/A probe into the AC and position the tip in the safe zone, using the technique described in the previous chapter.

- You will notice that if you push the eye *slightly* into depression, this gives you a better view of the lens matter under

the anterior capsule in the 5 o'clock region i.e. it allows you to see a little further under the iris in this area.

- Identify the anterior extent of cortex in this region. Advance the tip of the probe to this lens matter.

- Activate aspiration with the footpedal. As always, *use a low aspiration rate initially*

  → you should see the aspiration port engage the lens matter. If cortex is not engaged, increase the rate slightly

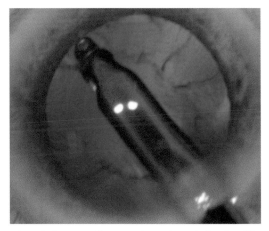

Fig 10.4 Targeting cortex at 5 o'clock with the straight I/A

  → *keep the aspiration port directed upwards so that it is visible at all times. Failure to do this results in an increased risk of accidentally engaging the capsule and causing a capsular tear*

  → if the cortex is positioned

peripherally in the capsular fornix, take care to avoid the anterior capsule, ensuring that you pass well beneath it

- If lens matter is engaged, it will occlude the port and you will hear a rise in pitch of the sound output, indicating that vacuum is being generated.

- With the lens matter engaged, maintain aspiration and draw the tip back to the safe zone

  → with a well dilated pupil you should be able to see cortex engaged in the aspiration port *before* drawing the I/A tip back

  → if you start to lose your hold on the cortex as you draw it to the centre, increase the aspiration rate as necessary to increase vacuum, provided the aspiration port is in view

  → if your hold on the cortex is lost completely, cease aspiration by returning to Position 1. You will need to repeat the above manoeuvre, first advancing the I/A tip to the cortex *before* activating aspiration, this time using a higher rate to generate more vacuum

- Once the tip is in the safe zone, depress the pedal further to aspirate the

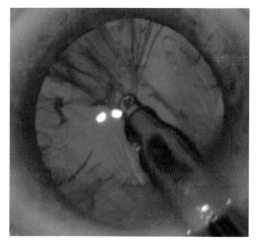

Fig 10.5 The aspiration port is drawn to the safe zone with cortex engaged

cortex. If necessary, the pedal *can be depressed fully* when the tip is in the safe zone

  → this combination of drawing the lens matter centrally and aspirating will cause a 'strip' of lens cortex to peel away from the capsule, beginning under the anterior capsule and extending around the equator to the posterior capsule

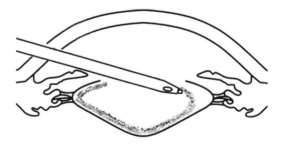

Fig 10.6 A strip of cortex is peeled away from the capsule

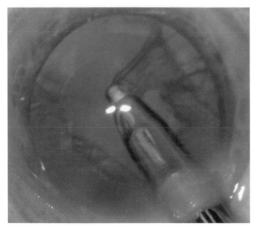

Fig 10.7 Aspirating a strip of cortex in the safe zone

the targeted area, so that it is positioned close to the capsular fornix, *before activating gentle aspiration. The aspiration port may now be out of view*

→ then withdraw the tip gently to see whether lens matter has been engaged – if not, cease aspiration and then repeat carefully with a slightly higher rate of aspiration

→ if cortex has been engaged, draw the tip back to the safe zone, increasing aspiration if necessary to maintain a grip

→ once the strip being peeled reaches the region of the central posterior capsule, it breaks off and is aspirated completely

• Now look for another area of cortex to target under the anterior capsule. Repeat the above manoeuvre.

Depending on the amount and distribution of cortex, it might not always be possible to see its anterior extent under the anterior capsule

→ you may be able to see cortex on the posterior capsule extending peripherally to the capsular fornix, but not be able to see any forward continuation under the anterior capsule

→ in such a situation you should advance the tip well underneath the anterior capsule in

Note
Cortex is engaged under the anterior capsule or in the equatorial fornix, as described above. Do not be tempted to engage cortex directly on the posterior capsule, as you will be more likely to engage the capsule itself and cause a tear.

A sign that the posterior capsule has been engaged is the appearance of characteristic stress lines in the PC, radiating out from the point where the capsule is engaged.

If you see or suspect that you have engaged the capsule, immediately STOP aspiration. The capsule may disengage straightaway. If not, *quickly proceed to activate fluid reflux* with the foot control (chapter 7), which should free the capsule from the aspiration port.

The 90° I/A

- In the sector shaded green in Fig 10.8, cortex should be cleared using the straight I/A. Work your way around this region, using the above technique repeatedly until the lens matter has been removed.

- When dealing with cortex in the sector shaded red, it is easier and *safer* to use the 90° I/A. The right-angled tip allows you to reach cortex under the anterior capsule in this region, while still keeping the aspiration port directed upwards.

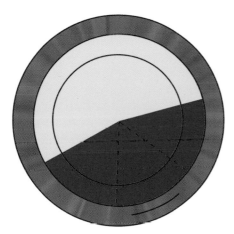

Fig 10.8 Use the straight I/A in the green sector; use the 90° I/A in the red sector; the sub-incisional region is demarcated (see later text)

- When inserting the 90° I/A, the tip enters the corneal section perpendicular to the wound. As the tip traverses the section, the instrument is rotated to bring the shaft perpendicular to the wound (i.e. you cannot simply push the

tip through the wound as you do with the straight I/A).

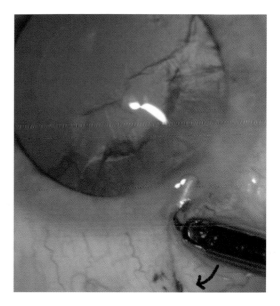

Fig 10.9 Rotating the 90° I/A tip through the corneal section. The cortex shown should all be removed using the 90° I/A

- The technique for aspirating lens matter is similar to that used with the straight I/A: the aspiration port is always directed upwards; the tip is passed under the anterior leaf of the capsule and cortex is engaged under direct vision if possible

  → however, instead of only drawing the instrument tip centrally as you do with the straight I/A, you can now *simultaneously rotate the aspiration port* towards the safe zone (Fig 10.10). Then increase the aspiration rate to aspirate the strip of cortex fully

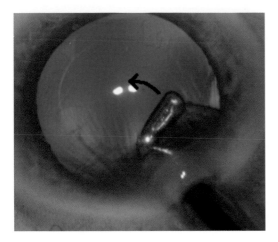

Fig 10.10 Rotation of the aspiration port towards the safe zone with cortex engaged

- You will find that you will need to hold the shaft more vertically than you do with the straight I/A in order to keep the aspiration port directed upwards at all times.

Sub-incisional cortex

Cortex immediately in front of the corneal section (demarcated in Fig 10.8) merits special attention. This is referred to as sub-incisional cortex, and is unique in that it is more difficult to see the peripheral and anterior extent of the lens matter in this region. This is because:

- the iris may obstruct more of your view

- the I/A probe itself obstructs part of your view

- corneal stress lines caused by the I/A shaft may obscure your view

It is usually possible to see whether or not lens matter is present here, but it is often not possible to see the anterior extent of the cortex which needs to be targeted with the aspiration port.

This is therefore a potentially dangerous area and extra caution should be exercised. It is the region where you are most likely to cause a capsular tear. Different strategies exist for dealing with cortex in this region, including making an additional paracentesis opposite the section so that the straight I/A can be used to access it.

However, we continue to use the 90° I/A with a modified technique:

Use the following technique for sub-incisional cortex

- To access sub-incisional cortex, the 90° I/A probe needs to be held close to vertical (as shown in Fig 10.11), with the aspiration port directed towards the targeted area. The pedal should be in Position 1 – irrigation only.

- If you are able to see the anterior extent of cortex in this region, engage it and proceed as described earlier.

- However, if you cannot, then advance the tip under the anterior leaf of the capsule towards the equatorial zone (Fig 10.11 & 10.12). The tip will usually *disappear from view* behind the iris (with average pupil dilatation)

  → *ensure that the tip passes deep to the anterior capsule*

→ ensure that the tip is peripheral enough to be close to the capsular fornix, without exerting stress on the rhexis margin or iris with the shaft of the I/A

- Activate aspiration: as always, *start with a low aspiration rate*

  → you may find that the targeted cortex disappears (into the aspiration port which is out of view), usually if it has been well hydrodissected

- If not, *cease aspiration* by returning to Position 1. *Rotate the I/A tip slowly into view to see whether any cortex has been engaged in the aspiration port* (cortex tends to stay stuck in the port if it has been properly engaged, even though aspiration is now off)

  → if there is lens matter engaged you can aspirate again, with a higher rate if necessary to maintain a good grip (because the port is now visible), while you rotate the tip towards the safe zone. Once in the safe zone you can aspirate maximally if necessary

  → however, if no cortex has been engaged, return the tip to the targeted area under the anterior capsule. Again activate aspiration, *this time using a slightly higher rate than before.* As previously, if the

cortex does not disappear into the aspiration port, cease aspiration and rotate the tip into view to see if any lens matter has been engaged (*footnote*)

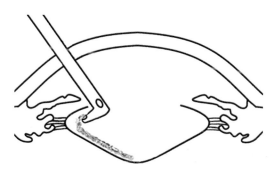

Fig 10.11 Sub-incisional cortex engaged out of view with the 90° I/A. Cease aspiration before rotating the tip into view

The principle is that when the aspiration port is out of view in the sub-incisional region, you should not move the I/A tip and aspirate simultaneously

  → the capsule and/or zonules are at greatest risk if the capsule has been engaged inadvertently with vacuum *and* the tip is then simultaneously moved

  → accidentally engaging the capsule with vacuum but a static aspiration port, or rotating with capsule engaged but without vacuum, are less likely to damage structures. *This is why aspiration is ceased before rotating the tip into view*

If repeated attempts to engage lens matter

do not bring success, try to target a different area of the sub-incisional cortex.

- Use the above method to complete the removal of all sub-incisional cortex.

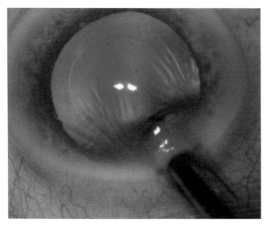

Fig 10.12 Accessing sub-incisional cortex with the 90° I/A

- You will need to remove the I/A probe from the eye for a complete view of the sub- incisional area to confirm that all the cortex has been cleared.

  The 90° I/A is removed in the reverse manner to which it is inserted → the tip must be rotated as it traverses the wound (with irrigation still running).

Potential pitfalls

Posterior capsular tear
The most important complication of I/A is a posterior capsular tear. This can allow vitreous to prolapse into the AC, requiring further intervention.

To minimise the risk of this:

- always keep the aspiration port directed upwards, away from the PC

- try to keep the aspiration port visible at all times. This is usually possible, except in the sub-incisional region

- if you need to engage cortex out of direct view, follow the technique described previously

  → *do not simultaneously aspirate and move the tip when the aspiration port is out of view*

- if you do engage capsule, stop aspirating *immediately*. If it does not disengage, activate reflux with the foot control (chapter 7).

Sometimes activating reflux does not cause release of the capsule:

  → it can then be helpful to pinch the aspiration line in your fingers and milk fluid towards the eye – this may release the capsule

Incomplete occlusion of the aspiration port
Sometimes you will find that only a fine, wispy strip of cortex becomes engaged in the aspiration port. This does not lead to complete occlusion of the port, so insufficient vacuum is created. As a result, you do not end up drawing any substantial lens matter to the safe zone

→ if this happens, return to Position 1 and advance the I/A tip slightly *more peripherally* in the targeted area than before

→ activate aspiration to see if a more substantial piece of cortex can be engaged

Shallow AC

If the AC is shallow, consider the same causes outlined in the section 'Shallow AC' on page 63. In such a case it is especially important that you do not inadvertently stop irrigation at any time:

→ *do not let the pedal come up out of Position 1*

→ you may wish to consider activating continuous irrigation (chapter 7)

If irrigation is interrupted the PC will move forwards and it is possible to damage it with the I/A tip.

Footnote

You should engage cortex with the lowest aspiration rate that is necessary to do so. Low rates are less likely to cause damage if the capsule is engaged accidentally. Therefore a particular aspiration rate is tried and the result observed. If your initial rate of aspiration fails to aspirate or engage anything, then you are justified in using a higher rate.

11
Preparing for Insertion of the IOL

Before the intraocular lens (IOL) can be inserted, the capsular bag needs to be re-formed by injecting viscoelastic. The corneal section usually needs to be widened, depending on the type of IOL, power of IOL, and the method of lens insertion you are using.

Method

On removal of the I/A probe from the anterior chamber, the capsular bag and the AC will shallow as the posterior capsule moves forwards (because there is no infusion of fluid to keep the AC formed).

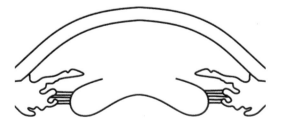

Fig 11.1 Shallowing of the AC and capsular bag as the PC moves forwards

• Before proceeding further, inspect the capsule to ensure there is no tear.

• In your right hand accept a syringe loaded with viscoelastic and mounted with a blunt cannula (Fig 4.1). Prime the syringe so that no air is contained. Use your left hand to provide stability as needed.

• Pass the tip of the cannula carefully through the corneal section into the AC, without pressing on the wound margins

→ *as soon as the tip is through the section inject some viscoelastic*

→ this pushes the posterior capsule backwards away from the cannula tip, so that you do not damage it

• *While still injecting slowly,* advance the cannula to a point just above the posterior capsule, in front of the capsulorhexis margin in the 5 o'clock region.

- Now slowly advance the tip under the anterior capsule towards the capsular fornix, *injecting viscoelastic gently as you go*

  → this pushes the posterior capsule backwards and the capsular bag begins to re-form in this area

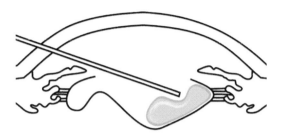

Fig 11.2 Capsular bag opposite the section re-forming

- Once the region of the bag opposite the corneal section has re-formed, withdraw the cannula to overlie the central posterior capsule and inject here *(footnote)*

  → the rest of the capsular bag will start to re-form

  → *you must see the posterior capsule pushed backwards by the viscoelastic, creating space for the IOL within the bag. You should see the bag distend as it is progressively filled*

- When you observe that the bag has been sufficiently re-formed to receive the IOL, stop injecting.

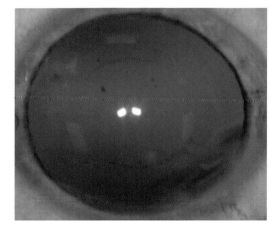

Fig 11.3 Capsular bag re-formed with viscoelastic

- Now draw the cannula back so that the tip is positioned just inside the AC, immediately in front of the section

  → inject a small amount of viscoelastic here

  → the purpose is to push the subincisional iris and anterior capsule backwards, away from the section, so that they are not damaged by the keratome when you widen the section

You should NOT overfill the bag and the rest of the AC with viscoelastic (footnote).

Widening the section

The keratome illustrated in Fig 3.1 yields

a corneal section with a width of 2.75mm. This will usually need to be widened, depending on the type and power of IOL, and the method of lens insertion you are using. Your supervisor should advise you what width of corneal section is required until you learn to judge this yourself.

To widen the section proceed as follows:

- With your left hand use notched forceps to stabilize the eye, as you do when initially making the corneal section (chapter 3).

- Use the keratome in your right hand. Pass *the tip* of the blade through the middle of the corneal section, such that the length of the blade now straddles the length of the corneal section

  → *keep the plane of the blade the same as the plane of the wound* during this manoeuvre, so that the blade passes cleanly through

- Now align the right cutting edge of the blade so that it is parallel with the right lateral margin of the corneal wound, as shown in Fig 11.4.

  Maintain the angle of the blade in the same plane as the wound.

- *In a single stroke,* exert gentle lateral pressure on the wound margin while the blade is *advanced* a few millimetres. This will widen the wound fractionally

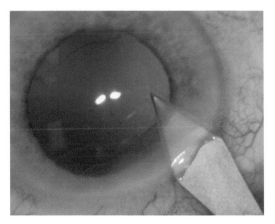

Fig 11.4 Alignment of the cutting edge parallel to the lateral wound margin

  → always incise the lateral wound margin on an inward stroke, as this maintains a constant tunnel length. *Avoid an in-and-out cutting action*

Measurement of the section

To determine the width of the section now, use callipers as shown in Fig 11.5. The callipers should be calibrated against a ruler before use. The tips of the callipers must abut the lateral margins of the wound.

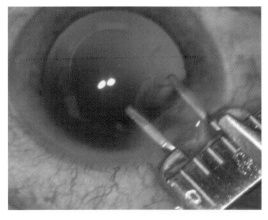

Fig 11.5 Osher callipers indicating a 3.2mm section width

- The section is widened as described above until the desired width is reached (it can also be extended to the left in a similar fashion).

- *It is better to have to repeat the sequence, re-measuring a few times, than to over-extend the wound unintentionally*

  → enlarging the wound more than necessary may prevent it from self- sealing. Therefore *use small increments* when first performing this step

  → with experience you will learn how much lateral pressure to exert with the keratome and how many cutting strokes are needed to achieve the required result more quickly

Potential pitfalls

PC tear

If you fail to inject viscoelastic ahead of the cannula as you advance it, you are at risk of tearing the posterior capsule

  → therefore start injecting slowly as soon as the tip enters the AC and inject whenever you advance the cannula

Loss of section architecture

When inserting the keratome through the section, be sure to follow the same planes that you used in the original construction of the section

  → if you angle the blade too steeply or shallowly, you may create a new false passage, compromising the seal of the section

Section too narrow/wide

If the section is too narrow, you will have difficulty inserting the IOL. Forcing a lens through a narrow section can result in uncontrolled, precipitous entry into the AC, with potential damage to structures.

If the section is too wide, it may not self-seal

  → measuring the wound and using small increments as described should prevent these problems

Footnotes

1. When filling the bag, viscoelastic is injected *distally before proximally*. This allows escape of BSS, which is displaced by the viscoelastic, through the section

  → if this sequence is not followed, then viscous viscoelastic may block the escape of BSS, causing a high IOP to develop during injection

2. If you use an injectable IOL, a small amount of viscoelastic is injected with the lens when you insert it. If you have mistakenly overfilled the AC with viscoelastic, this additional volume can cause a significant rise in IOP because the viscoelastic cannot escape when the section is plugged with the injector.

12

Insertion of the IOL

The intraocular lens (IOL) is inserted into the capsular bag via the corneal section. Either an injectable or a foldable lens is typically used. The technique of insertion depends on the type of IOL. We describe injectable lens insertion.

Often the injector will be loaded with the IOL by the assisting nurse and handed to you ready for use. In some units you may be expected to load the IOL yourself. Each type of injector is unique – you should familiarise yourself with the type used in your unit. The description which follows is by way of example and refers to one particular injection system – however, many of the principles are universal and apply irrespective of the system used.

The IOL & injector

- Before the IOL packaging is opened, the assisting nurse should confirm the type and power of lens that you have chosen. *Ensure that the lens is correct.*

- Fig 12.1 shows an injectable IOL,

which consists of an optic and two haptics. Note that the *haptics point in an anti-clockwise direction.*

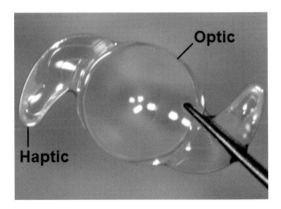

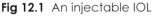

Fig 12.1 An injectable IOL

- After removing the IOL from its packaging, the lens must be kept with the correct side facing up

  → you must not turn the IOL back to front while handling it, as inserting the lens incorrectly may affect the optics

- Fig 12.2 shows a lens injector. In this injection system, the IOL is loaded into the cartridge.

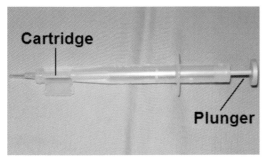

Fig 12.2 Lens injector

Loading the IOL into the cartridge

* Withdraw the plunger fully.

* Hold the injector horizontally in your left hand. The tip should face bevel down and the cartridge door must be open

 → the door tends to close due to elasticity of the plastic, so try to hold the injector in such a way that your left thumb and index finger keep it open (Fig 12.3)

* Fill the injector nozzle with viscoelastic and inject a trail of viscoelastic in each groove of the cartridge. Do not over-fill.

* Using non-toothed forceps, pick up the IOL from its packaging by *gently* grasping the optic. *Maintain its correct orientation.*

* Now, under the microscope, position the IOL in the cartridge as shown in Fig 12.3 (the haptic closer to the injector tip is called the leading haptic, while the one closer to the plunger is called the trailing haptic).

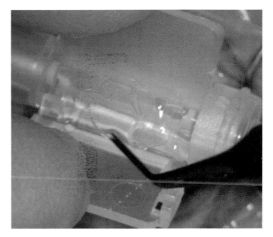

Fig 12.3 Lying the IOL down in the groove of the cartridge

* In order to close the door without catching any part of the IOL, the optic and haptics need to be pushed down into the groove of the cartridge

 → use forceps to press down on the optic as shown in Fig 12.4. This pushes it into the groove and also causes it to begin to fold

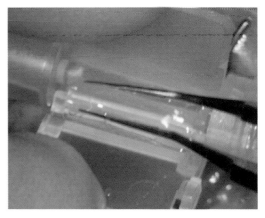

Fig 12.4 Use forceps to push the optic into the groove and induce a fold

→ use the forceps to induce a fold in each of the haptics and to push them down into the groove also

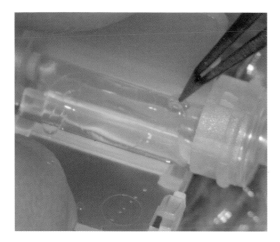

Fig 12.5 Pushing the leading haptic into the groove

• Close the door of the cartridge. It should close cleanly without resistance

   → closing the door rolls the lens up to allow injection

   → if the door fails to close easily, this may indicate that part of the IOL is trapped. *Do not attempt to force it closed as you may damage the IOL.* **You will have to reposition the lens, ensuring that the optic and haptics are properly pushed down into the groove**

• Check that the lens is freely mobile within the injector

→ push the plunger *just enough* to see if it causes movement of the IOL in the injector shaft without undue resistance

→ withdraw the plunger again: the IOL *should not move backwards with the plunger*. If it does, this implies that the trailing haptic has been caught

→ if you detect a problem you will need to re-open the cartridge door and reposition the IOL

Injecting the IOL

• Hold the injector in your left hand. Use your right hand to provide stability as needed.

• With the bevel of the injector tip facing downwards, position the tip immediately in front of the corneal section. The injector is orientated such that it points towards the centre of the capsular bag.

• Now gently depress the floor of the corneal section with the flat bevel, such that the wound opens slightly

   → this allows the tip to pass under the roof of the section

• Slide the tip forwards into the corneal section

   → you may need to wriggle the

tip gently to aid passage into the wound

→ the fit of the tip in the corneal section should be fairly snug (since the minimum required section width is used), so you will have to exert a *little* force

→ however, *if the tip will not enter the section, widen the wound fractionally*, rather than continue to push harder

→ the tip may pass fully into the AC, as in Fig 12.6, but this is not essential. It must, however, at least pass completely into the wound itself. Failure to achieve this may result in the IOL becoming stuck in the section when you attempt to inject

• Now orientate the injector such that the trajectory of the IOL is towards the distal capsular fornix

→ the IOL must be directed to pass beneath the anterior capsule opposite the section

• Gently push the plunger with the thumb of your right hand.

• Observe the progress of the lens as it is slowly injected. Adjust the orientation of the injector as necessary to ensure the IOL maintains the desired trajectory

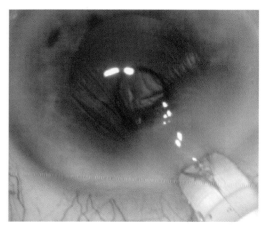

Fig 12.6 Injector tip positioned ready for IOL insertion

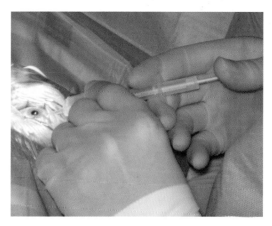

Fig 12.7 Injecting the IOL (a temporal corneal section was used in this case)

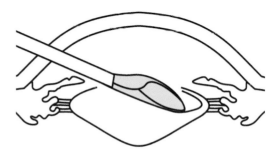

Fig 12.8 Correct trajectory during lens injection

→ as the IOL is injected, it begins to unfold

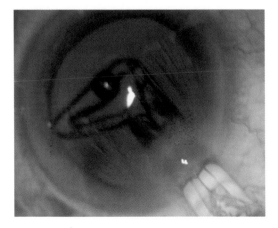

Fig 12.9 Unfolding of the IOL as it is injected – the leading haptic is entering the capsular bag

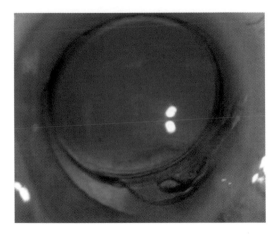

Fig 12.10 IOL post injection: the leading haptic is in the capsular fornix, the trailing haptic remains out of the bag

- Continue injecting until the IOL is completely free of the injector tip.

- Withdraw the injector *slowly*

  → if the lens is also drawn back when you start to withdraw the injector, then the IOL is not free of the tip

  → if this happens, draw back on the plunger a fraction and then re-inject. Repeating this action usually frees the IOL

The leading haptic should now be in/near the capsular fornix in the 5 o'clock region. The lens may have unfolded in such a way that the entire IOL is situated within the capsular bag, or the trailing haptic may still lie outside the bag, directed towards the corneal section.

Dialling in the IOL

If the entire IOL is not situated in the capsular bag after injection, you will need to dial/rotate it into position, so that both haptics end up in the bag.

- The haptics of the IOL are directed in an anti-clockwise direction. Therefore the IOL needs to be dialled in a *clockwise* direction.

- Rotating the IOL clockwise usually causes the trailing haptic to pass under the anterior leaf of the capsule, so that the IOL is then fully 'in the bag'.

To achieve this, a dialler (Fig 12.11) is used to manipulate the IOL.

This instrument can be used in any way you choose to move the IOL in a desired direction. Useful ways of gripping the IOL include:

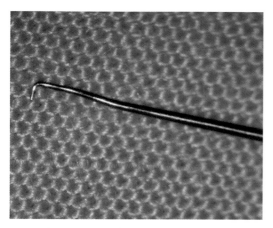

Fig 12.11 Sinskey hook (a dialler)

angle between the optic and trailing haptic allows good grip for a rotational force

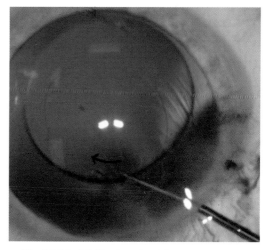

Fig 12.13 Dialler hooked into the angle between the optic and haptic to rotate the trailing haptic into the bag

(i) gently pressing down on the anterior surface of the optic with the tip of the dialler. If the tip is placed eccentrically on the optic, a rotational force can be applied using traction between the dialler and the IOL

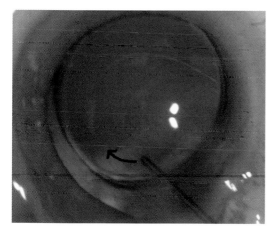

Fig 12.12 Rotational force being applied with the dialler

Method

- Insert the dialler into the AC via the corneal section using your right hand.

- Using techniques (i) or (ii) described above, begin by pushing the IOL gently downwards and further into the bag, such that *the leading haptic is convincingly in the capsular fornix.*

- Now rotate the IOL in a clockwise direction, using any of the techniques to gain a grip with the dialler

    → this tends to lead the trailing haptic under the anterior capsule so that it enters the bag

(ii) pushing against the rim of the optic or against a haptic

(iii) hooking the tip of the dialler into the

→ if you find that the trailing haptic pushes against the anterior leaf of the capsule but is reluctant to enter the bag, you may find it useful to push this haptic into the bag directly with the dialler

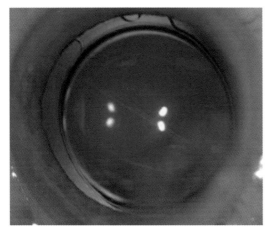

Fig 12.14 Optic and haptics 'in the bag' – the full circumference of the capsulorhexis should be seen in front of the optic

Potential pitfalls

Capsular bag not adequately re-formed
The capsular bag must be sufficiently re-formed with viscoelastic (chapter 11) to create space to accommodate the IOL. If you fail to re-form the bag adequately, you risk damaging the posterior capsule on injecting the lens. You may also find it difficult to dial the IOL into the bag.

Trapped haptic
If a haptic gets caught in the cartridge when you load the IOL, it may break during injection

→ *if you cannot demonstrate free movement of the IOL with gentle pressure on the plunger, or if the lens moves when you pull back on the plunger, reload it*

Difficulty inserting the injector
If you cannot pass the injector tip into the corneal section with gentle manipulation, extend the section width with the keratome.

Attempting to force the tip through the section may result in:

→ a precipitous, uncontrolled entry of the injector into the AC, with possible damage to the anterior segment

→ trauma to the wound margins, with the result that the section may not self-seal

→ a Descemet's membrane tear, where Descemet's membrane is stripped away at the inner aspect of the wound

Difficulty getting the trailing haptic into the bag
Measures to prevent this problem include:

→ initially ensuring that the capsular bag is well distended with viscoelastic to accommodate the IOL

→ pushing the leading haptic well into the capsular fornix *before* commencing rotation of the IOL

If the trailing haptic still proves to be a problem:

→ you may find it helpful to interrupt dialling the lens to inject more viscoelastic into the bag. This may create more space, allowing the haptic to enter the bag when you dial it again

→ if continued rotation fails to bring success, try pushing on the trailing haptic directly with the dialler to relocate it into the bag

13

Final Steps

After inserting the IOL, you need to remove the viscoelastic from the AC. You then re-form the AC with BSS and confirm that the wounds are self-sealing.

Removing the viscoelastic

Failure to remove the viscoelastic properly may result in elevated intraocular pressure post-operatively.

- Position the tip of the straight I/A close to the corneal section and activate irrigation.

- Pass the I/A tip into the AC

  → *the moment the tip enters the AC, immediately activate aspiration*[1]

- Position the aspiration port in the safe zone, *directed upwards*. Increase the aspiration rate → you will observe viscoelastic being displaced by BSS and aspirated

  → if necessary you may depress

the pedal fully with the aspiration port in the safe zone

  → maintaining high aspiration for *5 - 10 seconds* will remove most of the viscoelastic

- If you observe any viscoelastic anterior to the IOL after doing this, decrease the rate of aspiration and advance the tip carefully towards it in order to aspirate it.

At this point some viscoelastic may still be trapped behind the IOL. To facilitate its removal proceed as follows:

- Decrease the aspiration rate if it is maximal.

- Position the I/A tip such that it overlies a mid-peripheral part of the optic (Fig 13.1).

- Still aspirating, use the tip to push the underlying optic gently downwards, *so that the IOL is slightly tilted*

  → you may immediately see viscoelastic being displaced from behind the lens

→ if all is not removed, you can tilt the lens in another direction by gently pushing down on another eccentric part of the optic (the so called 'rock and roll' manoeuvre)

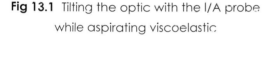

Fig 13.1 Tilting the optic with the I/A probe while aspirating viscoelastic

Take care to avoid engaging the capsulorhexis margin with the aspiration port during these manoeuvres.

- Once all the viscoelastic has been removed, cease aspiration and remove the I/A tip from the AC, with irrigation still running.

It may be difficult to see whether the viscoelastic has been removed from behind the IOL. Useful clues are:

→ often the optic shifts significantly as the viscoelastic

behind it is displaced by BSS

→ once the viscoelastic behind the IOL has been removed, the optic usually moves about a lot more within the bag as irrigation fluid circulates in the AC

→ the appearance of linear pleats in the posterior capsule is suggestive that the viscoelastic has been completely removed, though these will not always be seen

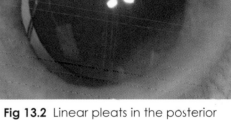

Fig 13.2 Linear pleats in the posterior capsule

AC formation

You now need to re-form the AC with BSS and confirm that both wounds are self-sealing, such that the eye maintains adequate intraocular pressure and AC depth.

- In your right hand accept a syringe filled with BSS, mounted with a blunt cannula. Use your left hand to aid stability as necessary.

- Insert the tip of the cannula into the *external* opening of the paracentesis (it should not pass all the way through the wound). The cannula should point towards the centre of the IOL.

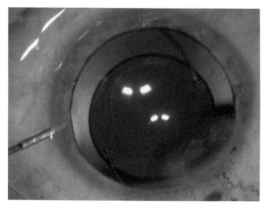

Fig 13.3 Cannula inserted into the external opening of the paracentesis

- *Gently* inject BSS while observing the AC, the corneal section and the paracentesis

    → you should see the AC deepen slightly

    → if there is leakage from the corneal section, this indicates that it is incompetent (not self-sealing). Suturing of the wound will be necessary

    → regurgitation of BSS via the paracentesis while injecting can be a reassuring sign. This implies that the corneal section is self-sealing. The leakage is usually due to the presence of the cannula in the external wound and ceases on its removal

- Remove the cannula tip *while still injecting*.

- Observe the AC for a few seconds

    → if the AC maintains its depth, this suggests the wounds are self-sealing

    → if the AC shallows significantly and/or the IOL moves forwards, at least one of the wounds is incompetent and will have to be sutured

- If AC depth is maintained, proceed to assess the intraocular pressure as follows:

    → rest the shaft of the cannula on the inferior sclera close to the limbus – this site is chosen to avoid distortion of the wounds

    → gently press down on the sclera: an indication of the IOP is gained from the amount of indentation caused by the cannula

    → you will learn what an acceptable IOP feels like through experience and advice from your supervisor *(footnote)*

- If the eye maintains an acceptable pressure and AC depth, then the wounds are

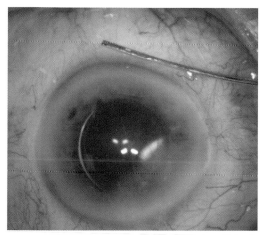

Fig 13.4 Assessing intraocular pressure

self-sealing and no intervention is required

If the eye is too hard

If you inject BSS too vigorously and the wounds are self-sealing, then the eye may end up too hard

> → reduce the IOP by using the cannula tip to depress the *floor* of the paracentesis briefly. This allows leakage of a small amount of BSS from the AC

> → reassess the IOP as before and release or re-inject BSS as necessary until an acceptable IOP results

If the eye is too soft

If the IOP is too low, you may have simply injected too little BSS at your first attempt

> → inject more BSS, watching the corneal wound closely for any leakage

> → if the eye still will not reach and maintain a satisfactory pressure, at least one of the wounds is incompetent and will need to be sutured

Identifying the site of leakage

It can be difficult to identify the site of leakage. This will usually be the corneal section, but occasionally the paracentesis is the problem. If you have not observed any obvious leakage as yet, the following may prove helpful:

- Use a spear swab to dry the conjunctiva immediately adjacent to the corneal section. This will make it easier to see whether there is leakage here.

- Inject BSS as before, observing the section.

- Again dry the area while looking for leakage

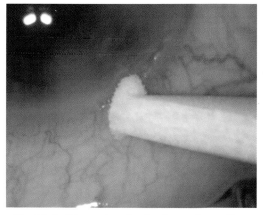

Fig 13.5 Observing for leakage from the corneal section

→ *touch the area only very lightly with the swab to avoid distorting the corneal section and inducing leakage*

- If no leakage is observed from the section, examine the paracentesis. Use the swab to dry the area around this wound after injecting BSS, observing for leakage.

- If either wound is shown to be incompetent, it will need to be sutured. Thereafter BSS must be injected to confirm that the wounds are sealing and that the eye maintains adequate pressure and AC depth.

Note
At this stage some surgeons hydrate the corneal stroma around the wounds. The resultant swelling of the cornea may cause sealing of an otherwise incompetent wound.

We do not perform this step. Our reasoning is that stromal hydration has a transient effect, so it is possible that a wound will again become incompetent later. If you are not satisfied that your wounds are self-sealing, it is safest to suture.

Subconjunctival injection

Many surgeons give a subconjunctival injection of antibiotic +/- steroid at this stage. Despite anaesthesia, this injection often stings: to avoid sudden movement, *advise the patient that s/he may feel brief discomfort.*

- In your right hand, accept a syringe mounted with a narrow gauge needle and primed with the antibiotic +/- steroid of choice.

- Using notched forceps in your left hand, gently grasp the bulbar conjunctiva in the inferior fornix, about 5mm from the limbus.

- Elevate the conjunctiva slightly away from the sclera.

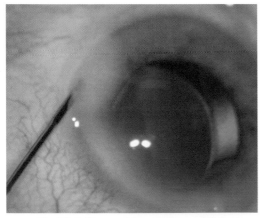

Fig 13.6 Stromal hydration of the paracentesis

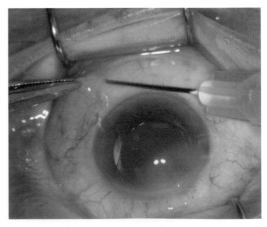

Fig 13.7 Subconjunctival injection

PHACO FUNDAMENTALS — A GUIDE FOR TRAINEE OPHTHALMIC SURGEONS

- With the bevel towards the eye, orientate the needle such that it is tangential to the scleral surface.

- *Avoiding vessels*, pierce the conjunctiva that is held tented up by the forceps. Inject to raise a bleb in the inferior fornix.

Note

Many surgeons choose to administer an intracameral antibiotic. A small volume is injected with a blunt cannula via the paracentesis, exactly as when injecting BSS to re-form the AC. Remember to assess the IOP again after injecting the antibiotic.

Final steps

- Move the microscope away from the patient.

- Inform the patient that you are about to remove the speculum and the adherent drape, which may be a little uncomfortable.

- To remove the speculum, first lift it forwards a little away from the globe

  → close it slightly by squeezing the two arms towards each other

  → then gently remove the inferior arm from under the lower lid, followed by the superior arm from under the upper lid

- Slowly peel the drape from the face. The patient's hair may have adhered to the drape, so look out for this and try to separate it carefully.

- When removing the drape, remember that the plastic pouch will contain fluid. Keep it orientated to prevent spillage onto yourself, the patient, or in the worst case, your supervisor!

- Use a moist swab to wipe away the povidone-iodine stain. Be very gentle around the eye, *taking care not to exert any pressure on the globe.*

- Dry the area with a dry swab.

- Tape a protective shield in place over the operated eye.

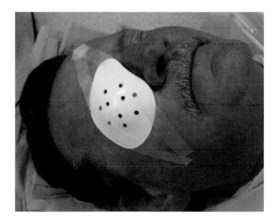

Fig 13.8 Protective shield taped in place

- Inform the patient that the operation is over and, if you have diligently followed the steps in this book, that all has all gone well!

Potential pitfalls

Failure to remove all the viscoelastic
This results in an increased risk of elevated IOP post-operatively. Therefore:

→ use a high aspiration rate in the safe zone for 5-10 seconds

→ look carefully for any sign of residual viscoelastic in the AC after this, especially behind the IOL

→ continue using the I/A as described previously until all is removed

Incompetent wounds
A leaking wound may lead to hypotony and its associated complications. Also, an incompetent wound may allow entry of ocular surface bacteria into the AC, increasing the risk of endophthalmitis

→ *if you are in any doubt that your wounds are self-sealing, it is safest to suture*

Footnotes
1. Irrigation without aspiration in an AC filled with viscoelastic may lead to a sudden rise in intraocular pressure.

2. It is useful to perform this manoeuvre before commencing the operation, after the eye is anaesthetised, to gauge what a normal pressure feels like.